Quick Referer W9-CDD-290
MANUAL OF CLINICAL PSYCHOPHARMACOLOGY
SECOND EDITION

Manual of Clinical Psychopharmacology
Second Edition

Alan F. Schatzberg, M.D.

*Professor of Psychiatry, Harvard Medical School,
Boston; Clinical Director, Massachusetts Mental
Health Center, Boston; and Director, Depression
Research Facility, McLean Hospital,
Belmont, Massachusetts*

Jonathan O. Cole, M.D.

*Director, Affective Disorders Program, McLean
Hospital, Belmont; and Lecturer in
Psychiatry, Harvard Medical School,
Boston, Massachusetts*

American
Psychiatric
Press, Inc

Washington, DC
London, England

Copyright © 1991 Alan F. Schatzberg and Jonathan O. Cole
First edition published 1986. Second edition 1991
ALL RIGHTS RESERVED
Manufactured in the United States of America on
acid-free paper.
94 93 92 91 6 5 4 3 2

American Psychiatric Press, Inc.
1400 K Street, N.W., Washington, DC 20005

Library of Congress Cataloging-in-Publication Data

Manual of clinical psychopharmacology, 2nd edition. / by Alan F.
Schatzberg, Jonathan O. Cole.
   p. cm.
   Includes bibliographical references.
   Includes index.
   ISBN 0-88048-318-0 (pbk.: alk. paper)
1. Mental illness—Chemotherapy. 2. Psychopharmacology.
3. Psychotropic Drugs. I. Schatzberg, Alan F. II. Cole, Jonathan O.
[DNLM: 1. Mental Disorders—drug therapy. 2. Psychotropic Drugs—
pharmacodynamics.
RC483.S37   1991
616.89'18
DNLM/DLC
for Library of Congress   86-1929
                                                                 CIP

British Library Cataloguing in Publication Data

A CIP record is available from the British Library

Contents

1 General Principles of Psychopharmacologic Treatment   1

2 Diagnosis and Classification   13

3 Antidepressants   31

4 Antipsychotic Drugs 85

5 | Mood Stabilizers 145

6　Antianxiety Agents　　185

12 Pharamacotherapy in Special Situations 313

List of Tables

List of Figures

Preface

In the first edition of the *Manual of Clinical Psychopharmacology* (1986) we set out to write a manual for the clinician that was both informative and easy to read. We have been extremely pleased by the response to the first edition. The many comments, thanks, questions, and suggestions we have received indicate that the book has been helpful to both practitioners and residents.

Although the first edition contained much then-current information about psychopharmacology and even data on medications that we anticipated would be released subsequent to publication, the mass of new material that has appeared since 1986 merits a second edition. We have added sections on new drugs (e.g., clozapine, selegiline, and clomipramine), expanded previous sections on important agents (e.g., fluoxetine, anticonvulsants in treating bipolar disorder), discussed in greater detail important treatment strategies for various disorders and situations (e.g., benzodiazepine discontinuation, obsessive-compulsive disorder), and updated other sections with the latest information from the literature and our clinical practice. Agents that may enter the market in the next 2–3 years are also reviewed (e.g., sertraline). Psychiatric syndromes addressed are now based on the more recent DSM-III-R classification and prevalence data on syndromes addressed are now presented.

Both the first and second editions of this book would not have been possible without the support, troubleshooting, and editorial guidance of Evelyn M. Stone. We, as well as many of our psychiatric colleagues around the United States, owe her a great debt for improving the quality of our work and the psychiatric literature as a whole. This book is dedicated to her.

Our wives and families deserve special thanks for allowing

us the time and effort needed on nights and weekends to complete this book. Linda Messier prepared and revised the manuscript and tables for publication.

This book grows primarily out of our work at McLean Hospital over the past 16 years and the recent work of one of us (A.F.S.) at the Massachusetts Mental Health Center (MMHC). Credit is due at McLean Hospital to Dr. Shervert H. Frazier, who recruited us, as well as to his successor, Dr. Steven Mirin. At MMHC, credit is due Dr. Miles F. Shore for his support and leadership of the Harvard Medical School department there. We are indebted to our colleagues, particularly our residents and staff in the Affective Disease Program at McLean Hospital and the Psychopharmacology Program at MMHC. We are also grateful to Lyn Dietrich of the McLean Hospital Services Library for her cheerful and skilled assistance with literature searches.

Last, the many patients we have tried to help over the years deserve much thanks. We hope that the next decade will bring even better treatments to ameliorate the suffering of psychiatric patients.

We hope readers will find this second edition as (if not more) useful as its predecessor. We look forward to feedback about any material contained herein and suggestions for later updates.

General Principles of Psychopharmacologic Treatment

Psychiatry has experienced a rapid metamorphosis over the past two decades in its methods of treatment. The move from a largely psychoanalytic orientation toward a more biological stance has not only radically changed our basic approaches to patients but also our own professional identities. For most psychiatrists, the transformation has not been easy. Keeping up with the ever-expanding information on biological theories, new laboratory tests, computerization, new medications, and new additional uses for old medications has in itself been a full-time occupation, one which often allows little time or energy to integrate current information into daily practice. Moreover, the proliferation of biological and psychopharmacologic information has occurred so rapidly that the task of integrating biological and psychotherapeutic approaches is made ever more difficult.

Some academics and practitioners would argue that psychopharmacologic approaches have become the essence of psychiatry, whereas others may insist that these drugs merely mask underlying diseases, work against conflict resolution, interfere with therapy, etc. Our impression has been that many, if not most, practitioners have developed more balanced, practical approaches which combine elements of both dynamic psychotherapy and psychopharmacology. In an odd way, academic psychiatry with its sometimes hypertrophied and polarized approaches has lagged *behind* clinical practice. Indeed, intuitively, we believe that psychiatry as a medical subspecialty will eventually incorporate aspects of psychosocial, psychobiological, and psychopharmacologic theories to form a truly "new psychiatry." One major reason for this is that although psychotropic drugs exert profound and beneficial effects on cognition, mood, and behavior, they often do not change the underlying disease process, which is frequently highly sensitive to intrapsychic, interpersonal, and psychosocial stressors. As a rule, beneficial outcomes can only be achieved by simultaneously reducing symptoms and promoting the capacity of the individual to adapt to the exigencies of his or her life. Strikingly, some practitioners of internal medicine have already come to embrace psychosocial principles to help such illnesses as hypertension, juvenile diabetes, and ulcer disease. Similarly, psychiatrists who overly embrace psychopharmacology as the be-all and end-all will probably find themselves in the same position as internists who feel prescribing thiazides is a simple solution to hypertensive illness. Conversely, practitioners of psychoanalysis should not expect that approach to "cure" or significantly reduce vegetative symptomatology in endogenously depressed patients. Rather they need to realize the potential benefits of alternative treatments—particularly psychotropic medication.

For practitioners who have not had extensive experience, a transition to a more pharmacologic practice is not without difficulties. A favorable clinical outcome after prescribing a psychotropic drug does reinforce confidence in psychopharmacologic approaches. Practically speaking, favorable outcomes can often be effected more quickly with a psychopharmacologic approach than with psychotherapy, so that confidence in psychopharmacology can be achieved readily.

Although this book is primarily a guide to psychopharmacology, its contents should not lead the reader to conclude that understanding how to select and prescribe psychotropic medications obviates the basic need to comprehensively evaluate and understand psychiatric patients. Our primary purpose is to provide the reader/practitioner with basic and practical information regarding the many classes of psychiatric medications. This book is written as a practical, usable clinical guide to the selection and prescription of appropriate drug therapies for individual patients, drawing on our own *clinical* experience as well as on the scientific literature. It is *not* a series of meticulously documented review papers, so individual statements in the text are often not individually referenced. However, each chapter is followed by a list of selected relevant articles and books for readers who wish to go beyond the material presented here.

GENERAL ADVICE

For the less experienced practitioner of psychopharmacology, a number of practical steps can be followed to assist in the development of skills and in the achievement of favorable outcomes.

Generally speaking, we recommend that practitioners concentrate first on one or two drugs per drug class and become fully familiar with how to use them (dosage, side effects, etc.). One's armamentarium of medication can then be widened over time and through further experience. The physician should have available some key resource materials—textbooks on psychopharmacology, *Physicians' Desk Reference* (PDR), etc. (Some helpful titles are found in the Suggested Reading List.) These can be supplemented with pharmacology newsletters, which provide useful current information. Moreover, practitioners should be familiar with a number of books directed at the lay audience that can help supplement information provided to patients (see Suggested Reading List). It is also a good idea to identify local psychopharmacologic consultants who can provide second opinions when needed, such as if patients fail to respond or if they experience severe side effects.

LEGAL/ETHICAL/ECONOMIC ISSUES

It seems prudent to discuss briefly a number of legal and ethical issues that have arisen in psychopharmacology. Since a comprehensive discussion of all of these is beyond the scope of this guide, the reader is referred elsewhere for specific information (see Suggested Reading List).

Informed consent has become an increasingly important issue in medicine. Standard medical practice has long called for informing patients of the risk-benefit ratio of various surgical and medical procedures. More recently, greater attention has been paid to the question of informed consent; for psychiatry, however, several key problems quickly arise. For one, psychiatrists must wrestle with the dilemma of evaluating the patient's capacity either to understand fully the benefits and risks of the medication prescribed or to interpret the provided information in a reflective and beneficial way. Obviously, this issue is particularly pressing in the psychotic patient, and legal guardianship may be required at times to effect adequate informed consent. Fortunately, these patients represent a minority of the average practitioner's patient population.

The paranoid, but competent, patient presents practical problems that are best overcome by creating a solid working relationship. Such patients are less commonly encountered than are highly anxious, obsessive, or agitated patients who are prone to adopt a phobic approach to medication. The practitioner at first glance may view informed consent in such cases as an insurmountable obstacle. Practically speaking, however, such patients will be anxious even if the practitioner does *not* inform them of side effects. Indeed, disclosing the facts often relieves their anxiety. It also connotes a respect for the severity of their illness and the need to mutually assume some risks.

Should the physician inform the patient of every side effect listed in PDR or merely highlight the most common ones? Some courts have judged that physicians may be liable if they do not tell the patient of every side effect. Practically speaking, most clinicians do not do so for several reasons, including the time involved and concern of unduly frightening the patient. The latter is particularly relevant when one reflects on the fact that package insert information lists virtually all side effects ever reported in drug trials, even if they were not due to the drug, plus side effects observed only or mainly with similar drugs. Still, we are impressed that patients not only have ready access to copies of PDR and consumer guides to medications but also commonly use them. In a sense, these practices begin to obviate the practitioner's perceived dilemma. Physicians need to enter into an open dialogue with all patients regarding the benefits and side effects of medication, even or particularly those patients who are self-taught. Patients who read PDR need to be informed of the relative probability of one or another side effect occurring. For example, patients should be made to realize that a dry mouth as the result of a tricyclic antidepressant is to be expected, but agranulocytosis or anaphylaxis is extremely rare. Our experience is that patients are reassured by the physician's belief (and hope) that these side effects will not be encountered. Recent package inserts often include tables comparing side effects in patients treated with a given drug to those observed with a placebo. This places the issues in a much better perspective.

Some physicians routinely hand to patients written materials (often a separate sheet for each medication) that spell out the medication's relative risks. This works well, but only if the practitioner feels comfortable with it and it becomes truly routine in his or her practice.

A particularly difficult problem revolves around the informed consent of risk for developing tardive dyskinesia, an unfortunate side reaction generally due to *long-term* treatment with antipsychotic medication (see Chapter 4). Tardive dyskinesia is a real risk in psychiatric practice. It affects some 14% of patients maintained on neuroleptic medication for 3 or more years and may be more common in patients with affective disorders than in those with schizophrenia. Thus, practitioners need to be particularly conservative in administering neuroleptics to patients who do not demonstrate frequent or chronic psychotic episodes. However, since chronic psychotic disorders do unfortunately exist, even prudent practice cannot eliminate the risk for tardive dyskinesia.

What should the physician tell the patient about tardive dyskinesia and when? Here a variety of approaches have been developed. One is to inform the patient and/or the family of the risk of tardive dyskinesia before prescribing neuroleptics. This may be too anxiety provoking and impractical, particularly for the acutely psychotic patient, since tardive dyskinesia generally is a long-term side effect and there is a pressing need to help compensate the patient quickly. Another approach is to broach the subject of the risk of tardive dyskinesia after approximately 4–6 weeks of treatment, before embarking on long-term or maintenance therapy. This seems more prudent to us.

Should one obtain written verification of informed consent? Here, too, different approaches have emerged. Some institutions and practitioners have adopted formal written informed consent. Others have adopted traditional verbal informed consent procedures and written documentation of the interchange in the patient's record. Still others have routinely provided the patient with additional written information regarding risks of tardive dyskinesia or other side effects (beyond PDR) but have not asked the patient to provide written informed consent. Each of these approaches has its advantages and its proponents. Currently, we recommend that practitioners and institutions adopt some formal documented disclosure of the risk of tardive dyskinesia and that they combine this with conservative administration of neuroleptics (both in terms of time and dosage) and a mutually cooperative undertaking of monitoring patients for the emergence of dyskinetic movements.

With the recent release of clozapine, psychiatrists should also seriously consider adopting a standard documented informed consent procedure for this potentially lethal but therapeutically unique drug. Patients incompetent to give informed consent should have a guardian who provides the consent.

In the past decade, physicians have been increasingly faced with the dilemma of prescribing standard drugs for indications that have not been approved by the U.S. Food and Drug Administration (FDA) or at doses that are higher than those recommended in PDR. In some instances, drugs can be misprescribed, and this can obviously be dangerous. In many others, considerable clinical or research data have emerged pointing to potentially great benefits to many patients, but package insert information may not have been changed because of economic or regulatory factors. For example, imipramine today is commonly prescribed to both outpatients and inpatients at doses of 300 mg/day. Still, the package insert states that outpatients should not receive more than 225 mg/day. In part, this reflects the fact that approved dosage regimens were determined on the basis of data generated many years ago when a greater proportion of seriously depressed patients were treated as inpatients and before the application of plasma levels (see Chapter 3). It is unlikely that the package insert will be changed. Additional studies to further document the efficacy and safety of higher dosages would be too costly for drug manufacturers, who can no longer hope to recoup the costs of such study since the patent for the drug may have long since expired. One pharmaceutical manufacturer several years ago applied for and was granted FDA approval to raise the maximum daily dose of its nortriptyline compound (Pamelor) from 100 to 150 mg/day. A manufacturer of an identical nortriptyline compound—Aventyl—did not, and this product enjoys only a 100-mg maximum daily dose. Thus, we have on the U.S. market two identical nortriptylines with different maximum daily doses.

Examples of so-called nonapproved uses include the use of imipramine and phenelzine for patients with agoraphobia or panic disorder or the use of carbamazepine in manic-depressive illness. There is a growing body of data that these drugs are effective, but market conditions and regulatory guidelines may result in some, or even all, of these drugs not being granted official new indications. Is the practitioner at legal risk in prescribing these drugs? Generally, the American Medical Association and FDA have taken the position that the use of any marketed drug for "nonapproved" indications or at higher dosages for individual patients is within the purview of the clinician. PDR is not an official textbook of medical practice but rather a compendium of drug information for marketing purposes. It sets limitations on what pharmaceutical companies can claim for their products. Malpractice is based on failure to practice within community norms. Still, many clinicians will not easily accept the potential risk of being sued—even if such a suit may have little merit—by a patient who experiences an untoward reaction to a standard drug used for a "nonapproved" indication or to a dose of drug that is higher than the recommended maximum dose.

What are the solutions? Until various forces (both patients and physicians) come to the fore to effect a change in the system for widening indications or for maximum doses, each clinician must decide whether he or she wishes to assume the risk. However, while clinicians may attempt to opt for a conservative approach, they will at some point encounter patients who will require alternative treatments. One possible aid may be to acquire outside consultation from more expert psychopharmacologists or from other practitioners in the community. Another is to explain the scope of the problem to patients, providing them with available published reports on positive benefits, and documenting this in their records. Some physicians will ask for written documentation that the patient has been informed. In the end, there are no simple solutions, and the physician will at some point be faced with this problem.

There is another issue that faces psychiatrists treating treatment-resistant patients. There are numerous antidepressant and antipsychotic drugs available in Canada or in European countries. Canadian drugstores had been mailing clomipramine regularly to the United States after receiving a prescription (and a check) from the patient. With the growth of pressure from patients with acquired immunodeficiency syndrome (AIDS), our FDA appears to view favorably (or at least passively) the importation of a 3-month supply of drugs not available in the United States for the treatment of an individual patient. With the recent release of clomipramine, the only semi-antidepressant drug available in Canada but not in the United States is L-tryptophan, but well-established drugs such as mianserin, older monoamine oxidase inhibitors (iproniazid, nialamide), and newer drugs such as fluvoxamine are available in Europe, and psychiatrists may be able to obtain them through colleagues, friends, or relatives there.

Many patients received Canadian clomipramine for years without our ever hearing of a malpractice suit. Nevertheless, the possibility exists. In 1987, Dr. Robert Dupont wrote to the American Psychiatric Association's malpractice insurers to ask whether his malpractice insurance would cover him were he to be sued for an adverse effect from clomipramine imported from Canada. He was told he would not be covered. Other plans do cover such situations. Psychiatrists wishing to treat patients with imported drugs not approved in the United States should consider the risks to themselves as well as to their patients.

Cost containment has led many health plans to prefer generic compounds over proprietary drugs. We are frequently asked about the advisability of prescribing generic compounds. For many years, the FDA has only required that a manufacturer demonstrate that a given dose of a compound will produce blood levels within 20–30% of the proprietary form. Obviously, for some medications (e.g., tricyclic antidepressants) this can prove problematic. Lower blood levels of a tricyclic antidepressant may result in the patient not achieving therapeutic levels when treated with traditional doses. Moreover, switching to an equivalent dose of a generic compound in patients who have responded to a given dosage of a standard antidepressant may result in loss of therapeutic effect. Differences between generic and proprietary forms can go in both directions. The generic form could lead to higher, potentially toxic blood levels.

As this second edition was being written, the FDA ordered that a number of generic benzodiazepine compounds be removed from the market because they had fallen below minimum standards. Thus, quality control of the manufacturing of generic compounds may not necessarily meet acceptable standards. However, there may be significant variability between different batches of the same proprietary drug as well. New regulations have been proposed to bring generic compounds closer to equivalency with their proprietary counterparts.

We currently recommend that physicians start their patients on proprietary compounds and adjust dosages until therapeutic benefit has been achieved and side effects have been limited. Generic compounds can be used for maintenance therapy. Blood levels for the specific medication should be obtained while the patient is still being treated with the proprietary compound, before switching to the generic, and rechecked while the patient is on the equivalent dose of the generic if the patient loses therapeutic benefit or experiences side effects.

Another consequence of cost containment is health plans' insistence that patients obtain 3-month supplies of medications, generally during maintenance therapy. Obviously, in patients with a history of abuse of medications or suicidal behavior, this can prove problematic.

We recommend using good clinical sense in deciding how many pills or capsules to prescribe. Frequently, local pharmacies will work with physicians and patients to come to a clinically and economically sound compromise (e.g., agreeing to hold supplies in patients' names but dispensing in 1- to 2-week quantities).

In this book, we have attempted to provide practical information regarding many different psychotropic drugs. Information regarding dosages is for adult patients (ages 18–60 years) unless otherwise noted. We have included information derived from our reading of the psychiatric literature as well as from our own clinical practice. We have attempted to indicate, wherever possible, those uses that officially have not been approved by the FDA for marketing purposes, but we have also attempted to provide the readers with sufficient data so that they can decide whether or how they may wish to prescribe specific drugs. In so doing, we are not endorsing their use but are realistically attempting to place a drug in its proper perspective. We believe "real-world" psychiatric practice dictates that we provide the practitioner with information based on either the scientific literature or on common clinical use, even though a drug's indications may not yet have been changed or—perhaps because of economic reasons—may never be changed.

Bibliography

Applebaum PS: Legal and ethical aspects of psychopharmacologic practice, in Clinical Psychopharmacology, 2nd Edition. Edited by Bernstein JC. Boston, MA, Wright PSG, 1984

Erickson SH, Bergman JJ, Schneeweiss R, et al: The use of drugs for unlabeled indications. JAMA 243:1543–1546, 1980

The FDA Does Not Approve Uses of Drugs (editorial). JAMA 252:1054–1055, 1984

Gutheil TG: Liability issues and malpractice prevention, in Handbook of Clinical Psychopharmacology. Edited by Tupin JP, Shader RI, Harnett DS. Northvale, NJ, Jason Aronson, 1988, pp 439–453

Nonapproved uses of FDA-approved drugs. JAMA 211:1705, 1970

Use of approved drugs for unlabeled indications. FDA Drug Bulletin, April 1982

Use of drug for unapproved indications: your legal responsibility. FDA Drug Bulletin, October 1972

Diagnosis and Classification

2

In the past decade, psychiatry has paid greater attention to rigorous diagnosis and classification, as evidenced by the 1980 publication of the then forward-thinking *Diagnostic and Statistical Manual of Mental Disorders, Third Edition* (DSM-III) and its subsequent revision in 1987, DSM-III-R. Much of this attention has been sparked by advances in the biology and treatment of various psychiatric disorders, making precise diagnosis ever more important. For example, the response of many patients diagnosed with bipolar (manic-depressive) illness to lithium carbonate fostered the adoption of rigorous efforts to discriminate between manic-depressive illness and schizophrenia, resulting in a change of diagnosis for many patients and subsequent alterations in their treatment.

Approaches to psychopharmacologic treatment are often based on trying to match a given treatment or a combination of treatments with a specific diagnosis. Although this approach represents the ideal, it is only effective in approximately 60% of patients because

- Many patients have a disorder that is not easily classified.
- Some patients with a seemingly classic disorder may not respond to a traditional drug.
- Increasingly, various drugs have been shown to exert wider actions than their drug class eponym (e.g., anticonvulsants) suggests.

Thus, the clinician must combine the "ideal" paradigm with a more flexible approach—one that attempts to match a given treatment with various clusters of symptoms rather than with an overall syndrome. The danger of this approach, however, is that—if carried too far—it can result in unhealthy polypharmacy. Obviously, the clinician must attempt to develop a general strategy for matching a range of specific treatments to patients with particular diagnoses or symptoms.

A sound general philosophy is to ascertain whether patients meet symptom criteria for a disorder (e.g., major depression with melancholia) that is generally thought to commonly respond to a given class of drug or treatment (e.g., tricyclic antidepressants) and then to prescribe classic representatives of the given drug class (e.g., imipramine). This can later be followed by a shift to less traditional medications if initial trials do not prove to be effective. Such an approach is sound overall; however, clinicians must be aware that diagnostic classifications have inherent limitations that can be misleading. For example, it was our impression that many patients who had been diagnosed with DSM-III major depression did not respond to antidepressant drugs, often requiring some form of psychotherapy (e.g., interpersonal psychotherapy or cognitive therapy). In part we believed this was due to the limited number and type of symptoms that were required for a disorder to be diagnosed as major depression. Indeed, although major depression is commonly mistaken as representing an endogenous type of depressive illness, in fact—historically and practically speaking—endogenous depression (which is classically believed to respond to tricyclic antidepressants) is only a subtype of major depression. DSM-III-R criteria for major depression are somewhat tighter than they were in DSM-III, suggesting that this problem may have been obviated to some degree.

Although comprehensive discussion of psychiatric classification is beyond the scope of this monograph, it is useful to review the DSM-III and DSM-III-R systems and the prevalence rates for major categories of adult psychiatric disorders and to highlight which types of psychopharmacologic agents often prove most beneficial in each category. Prevalence rates provided in this chapter are based primarily on recent reports from the Epidemiologic Catchment Area (ECA) program. Table 2-1 summarizes DSM-III-R disorders described in this chapter.

MOOD DISORDERS

Mood disorders by definition are pathological affective states. In DSM-III, these disorders were termed *affective disorders.* They were divided into "major affective" and "other specific" subcategories that were then further broken down along a bipolar versus unipolar dimension. In DSM-III-R, disorders are initially divided into bipolar and depressive disorders that are then further subdivided into distinct entities. Also, the severity of the disorder and the degree of psychosocial precipitants and seasonal pattern are specified.

Bipolar Disorders

Bipolar disorders are subdivided into bipolar disorder (mixed, manic, or depressed), cyclothymia, and bipolar disorder not otherwise specified (NOS). To be diagnosed as having *bipolar disorder* (manic-depressive illness), the patient must currently meet criteria for hypomania or mania or must have had a prior episode that met criteria for either of these syndromes. The current episode is further categorized according to

Table 2-1.   DSM-III-R diagnoses addressed

I. *Mood Disorders*
   A. Bipolar disorders
   B. Depressive disorders
      1. Major depression
      2. Dysthymia

II. *Schizophrenic Disorders*

III. *Psychotic Disorders Not Elsewhere Classified*
   A. Schizophreniform
   B. Schizoaffective

IV. *Anxiety Disorders*
   A. Simple phobias
   B. Social phobias
   C. Agoraphobia with or without panic attacks
   D. Panic disorder
   E. Generalized anxiety disorder
   F. Obsessive-compulsive disorder
   G. Posttraumatic stress disorder

V. *Somatoform Disorders*
   A. Psychogenic pain disorder

VI. *Personality Disorders*
   A. Borderline
   B. Paranoid
   C. Antisocial

VII. *Psychoactive Substance Use Disorders*
   A. Alcohol and drug abuse
   B. Alcohol and drug dependence

VIII. *Disorders of Childhood and Adolescence*
   A. Attention-deficit hyperactivity disorder
   B. Bulimia nervosa

whether the patient is manic, depressed, or experiencing a mixed affect state.

Criteria for mania include a distinct period of persistently elevated or irritable mood sufficient to cause harm or to result in hospitalization. At least three of seven symptoms need to be included (four if only irritability is present): increase in activity, increased speaking, flight of ideas, inflated self-esteem, decreased need for sleep, distractibility, and overinvolvement in high-risk activities (e.g., spending sprees, reckless driving). Since in DSM-III only a limited number of symptoms needed to be present and for only a relatively brief period (1 week), some investigators and clinicians argued that the criteria were too broad. In DSM-III-R, the minimum period for presence of symptoms is not specified; rather, only that a distinct period is required. However, if the episode is not severe enough to affect performance or result in hospitalization, the episode is termed *hypomania* and the patient is diagnosed as bipolar disorder NOS. This disorder is similar to bipolar II disorder using the Research Diagnostic Criteria (RDC). The 6-month and lifetime prevalence rates of mania in the general population are approximately 0.5 and 0.8%.

The classic psychopharmacologic treatment approach for overall mood stabilization of these disorders involves lithium carbonate or lithium citrate; recently, carbamazepine, valproic acid, and clonazepam have also been shown to have mood-stabilizing effects, most prominently in acute mania (see Chapter 5). Treatment of acute hypomania or mania includes the mood-stabilizing drugs noted above as well as antipsychotic, neuroleptic agents and sedative-hypnotics for sleep. Treatment of bipolar depression often requires combining lithium with treatments used for major depression (see below).

As described above, the major strides made toward a wider redefinition of bipolar manic states have undoubtedly resulted in more patients receiving lithium carbonate. The potential benefit to many patients in this broadening of diagnoses must be weighed against a procrustean tendency to overdiagnose the disorder in order to justify lithium treatment. Not uncommonly, clinicians see patients who have a chronic disorder that was once termed schizophrenia but has now been rediagnosed as either a bipolar manic-depressive or schizoaffective illness. Unfortunately, many such patients do not respond to lithium, pointing to certain inherent limitations in overbroadening this category.

Cyclothymic disorder is a more chronic and less severe illness than bipolar disorder. A 2-year course with repeated episodes of mild mood cycles is required to meet criteria for this disorder. Patients may begin with a cyclothymic disorder but develop superimposed bipolar disorder or bipolar disorder NOS. Many investigators claim that lithium carbonate is of benefit to some patients with cyclothymic disorder.

Depressive Disorders

Major depressive episode is by definition a *unipolar disorder* if the patient does not have a history of hypomania or mania (i.e., a bipolar disorder). Six-month and lifetime prevalence rates are 3% and 6%, respectively, and women are more commonly affected than men. Criteria for a major depressive episode consist of a variety of signs and symptoms, including appetite disturbance, sleep disturbance, psychomotor retardation or agitation, suicidality, decreased interest in life, and guilt. Obviously, many of these symptoms are those that European and American investigators have used to describe "endogenous depression." Unfortunately, a patient may meet criteria for a major depressive episode without demonstrating much in the way of endogenous symptoms. In DSM-III, only four symptoms were required to meet the diagnosis of major depressive episode; DSM-III-R requires five symptoms. However, only a 2-week duration of symptoms is needed to meet criteria in both systems.

A subtype of major depression ("with melancholia") more closely resembles "endogenous depression." In DSM-III-R, criteria for this subtype have been modified to require presence of five of nine features: distinct loss of pleasure in activities, lack of reactivity to pleasurable stimuli, diurnal variation, marked psychomotor retardation or agitation, early morning awakening, significant weight loss, no premorbid personality disorder, complete recovery from previous major depressive episode, and previous good response to antidepressants. It is not yet clear whether major depression with melancholia will fully approximate endogenous depression because 1) similarly brief time periods are applied as in major depression, and 2) previous response to somatic treatments and previous recoveries may prove to be unrelated to melancholia specifically. Further research will hopefully lead to even better phenomenologic definition of this disorder.

An important subtype of major depressive episode—"major depressive episode with psychotic features"—by definition involves delusional thinking as evidenced by guilty or nihilistic delusions, hallucinations, and even communicative incompetence. This specific disorder represents some 8–30% of all major depressions.

Primary treatments for major depression include tricyclic antidepressants (TCAs), monoamine oxidase inhibitors (MAOIs), electroconvulsive therapy (ECT), trazodone, and bupropion. Secondary treatments are lithium carbonate and the triazolobenzodiazepine alprazolam. Major depressive episode with psychotic features often reacts poorly to TCAs alone; it may require a combination of antidepressants and phenothiazines or ECT.

Dysthymic disorder (depressive neurosis) is a more chronic condition whose symptoms by definition are not severe enough to meet criteria for major depression. In DSM-III, the criteria for dysthymic disorder were broad, and a number of the symptom criteria were not specifically those of depression, e.g., anxiety, irritability, and obsessionality. In DSM-III-R, two of six depressive symptoms are required: appetite disturbance, sleep disturbance, fatigue, decreased self-esteem, decreased concentration or indecisiveness, and hopelessness. Six-month and lifetime prevalences for dysthymic disorder are approximately 3%. There is little evidence that antidepressants are truly effective in this condition; however, if the condition is severe enough, they may prove helpful. Probably related to dysthymic disorder (but not identical to it) is "atypical depression," a nonendogenous depressive illness with pronounced anxiety, for which English psychiatrists have long advocated treatment with MAOIs.

SCHIZOPHRENIC DISORDERS

Schizophrenic disorders are primarily disorders of cognition and thinking—in contrast to disorders of mood. These syndromes are heterogeneous with multiple subtypes described in DSM-III. Of particular importance in these conditions are delusions (often persecutory in nature), prominent and persistent hallucinations (primarily auditory), loose associations, catatonia, and flat or inappropriate affect.

Further, the illness's course is chronic (at least 6 months) and often deteriorating, and the patient commonly shows social isolation and withdrawal. Six-month and lifetime prevalence rates of schizophrenic disorders are 0.8 and 1.3%, respectively. Primary treatments are the neuroleptic antipsychotics, which include, for example, phenothiazines, butyrophenones, and thioxanthenes. Clozapine, an atypical neuroleptic, shows considerable promise in refractory patients. Some investigators have reported limited benefit with lithium. The efficacy of tricyclics for some anergic/depressed schizophrenic patients has also been demonstrated, interestingly, with a relatively low incidence of worsening of psychosis.

Schizophreniform and schizoaffective disorders are subsumed under "psychotic disorders not elsewhere classified." *Schizophreniform disorders* differ from schizophrenia only in duration of illness—lasting from 2 weeks to 6 months. This is a rarer disorder with 6-month and lifetime prevalence rates of 0.1%. Acute treatment for this condition generally involves neuroleptics. *Schizoaffective disorder* is used when the history is not clear enough to allow for a more precise diagnosis (e.g., bipolar disorder, schizophrenia). For example, some patients with an episodic mood disorder and a significant thought disorder as seen in schizophrenia would receive this diagnosis. Also, a patient with residual evidence of psychosis when in "remission" from a mood disorder may also receive this diagnosis. Such patients often receive the most complex drug regimens in a valiant effort to control a mix of affective, schizophrenic, and even anxiety symptoms.

ANXIETY DISORDERS

The DSM-III classification of anxiety disorders was radically different from its DSM-II predecessor, and DSM-III-R has elaborated further on this approach.

Anxiety in DSM-III was divided into two main categories: phobias and anxiety states. Phobias were subdivided into simple (e.g., animals, storms), social (interpersonal situations, public speaking, etc.), and agoraphobia (fear of open spaces or of being alone) with or without panic attacks. The anxiety states were divided into generalized anxiety disorder, panic disorder, posttraumatic stress disorder, and obsessive-compulsive disorder. In DSM-III-R, the broad distinction between phobias and anxiety states has been dropped. Instead, anxiety disorders are divided into eight subtypes. In addition, panic disorder has become even more prominent, with agoraphobia with panic attacks now being subsumed under panic disorder.

Whereas considerable progress in classifying anxiety is reflected in DSM-III-R, a great deal of confusion and debate still remains. This is particularly evident in the lingering questions of how to subdivide the group of disorders included under agoraphobia, agoraphobia with panic attacks, panic disorder, social phobia, and generalized anxiety disorder.

The *simple phobias* include encapsulated fears and avoidance of specific stimuli (e.g., heights, animals, closed spaces). Animal phobias are almost exclusively found in females and generally begin in childhood. The 6-month and lifetime prevalence rates of simple phobias are extremely high—approximately 8 and 13%, respectively. The conditions are generally treated with behavior therapy.

Social phobias involve intense and undue fears and avoidance of interpersonal interactions, urinating in public bathrooms, etc. They occur in both sexes and begin in late adolescence and early adulthood.

Agoraphobia—the fear of being alone or in open spaces (e.g., supermarkets or shopping malls)—has attracted increasing attention in recent years, as particularly seen in numerous psychopharmacologic and psychotherapeutic studies on DSM-III agoraphobia with panic attacks. As indicated above, in DSM-III-R such patients are labeled as having panic disorder with agoraphobia. When frank panic attacks are not present, a diagnosis of agoraphobia without panic is made. Such patients may experience partial panic attacks—"limited symptom attacks." Some investigators have argued that agoraphobia does not occur without significant limited symptom or panic attacks; however, a recent analysis of ECA data indicates that agoraphobia without frank panic attacks is far more common than was once thought.

Agoraphobia is far more common in women than in men, and the mean age at onset is the late 20s. The lifetime prevalence rate of agoraphobia is approximately 4%. The disorder can be disabling since patients may markedly constrict their daily activities. The phobic aspects may be treated via behavior therapy or psychotherapy. Acute symptomatic relief may be best effected by using benzodiazepines. Criteria for DSM-III-R *panic disorder* are somewhat more rigorous than they were in DSM-III. Panic disorder is characterized by at least four episodes of panic—acute, almost incapacitating anxiety—in a 4-week period or one or more attacks, followed by persistent fear (lasting at least 1 month) of having another attack. These attacks are characterized by at least 4 of 13 symptoms including dyspnea, chest discomfort, palpitations, lightheadedness, sense of dread, hot and cold flashes, sweating, faintness, etc. If they are associated with agoraphobia, a diagnosis of panic disorder with agoraphobia is made. The 6-month and lifetime prevalence rates of panic disorder are approximately 0.8 and 1.1%, respectively, and the disorder is more common in women than in men.

There was considerable debate whether there was a meaningful difference between panic and agoraphobia with panic in DSM-III, some investigators having posited that agoraphobia was a form of end-stage, avoidant behavior to defend against possible panic attacks. DSM-III-R has in part adopted this position but still retains agoraphobia without panic as a separate entity. Other investigators have even argued that generalized anxiety disorder is an end-stage generalization of earlier panic symptoms, so-called endogenous anxiety. Since patients who have agoraphobia with panic respond to alprazolam, imipramine, and phenelzine, it is generally presumed that patients with panic disorder will respond similarly.

In DSM-III, *generalized anxiety disorder* was characterized by persistent anxiety of at least 1 month. In DSM-III-R, anxiety symptoms must be generally present for at least 6 months. Symptoms are grouped under motor tension—shakiness, tension, trembling, etc.; autonomic hyperactivity—sweating, heart pounding, cold hands, etc.; and vigilance and scanning—difficulty in concentration, insomnia, irritability, etc. The disorder is more common in women than in men. Earlier studies pointed to prevalence rates ranging between 2 and 6%. Prevalence rates of this newly defined DSM-III-R diagnosis have not been well established. Some investigators believe the current criteria will make diagnosis of generalized anxiety disorder extremely rare, but a recent analysis of ECA data suggests this is not the case, and prevalence rates of 2.5% have been reported.

Various drug classes may be effective in treating generalized anxiety disorder, including benzodiazepines, buspirone, barbiturates, antihistamines, phenothiazines, and meprobamate. However, of these medications, benzodiazepines are overwhelmingly the most commonly prescribed. Recently, TCAs have also been shown to be effective in treating this disorder.

Obsessive-compulsive disorder is characterized by obsessions and compulsions producing significant distress. Obsessions are recurrent, persistent ideas and thoughts that are ego-dystonic and that individuals attempt to suppress or neutralize. Compulsions are defined in DSM-III-R as "repetitive, purposeful, and intentional behaviors that are performed in response to an obsession, according to certain rules, or in a stereotyped fashion." The disorder is more common in women than in men, and 6-month and lifetime prevalence rates are 1.5 and 2.5%, respectively. Often, patients with pronounced obsessive-compulsive symptoms are at closer inspection found to meet criteria for major depression. Preliminary studies suggest that clomipramine, a TCA with pronounced serotonin reuptake blocking properties, is effective in this condition. Preliminary data suggest that the newer specific serotonin reuptake blockers (e.g., fluoxetine) may also be effective in this condition. Other TCAs and MAOIs have also been found, in limited studies, to be somewhat effective.

Posttraumatic stress disorder has come under increased attention since the Vietnam War. The disorder is characterized by the existence of a recognizable stressor that would be inferred to potentially evoke distress in most individuals. Previous trauma is reexperienced via recurrent recollections or dreams of the event or a sudden sense that the event is recurring. Often these patients demonstrate decreased responsiveness or involvement with the external world. Common symptoms include startle responses, memory or concentration problems, sleep disturbance, guilt about surviving, avoidance of stimuli that mimic or simulate the event, and recrudescence of symptoms upon exposure to stimuli. Although the disorder has achieved wide popular interest because of the political aspects of the war in Vietnam, similar disorders, such as traumatic war neurosis in World War II pilots, have long been known in the literature. The prevalence of the disorder is unclear. Also, psychopharmacologic treatment has not been well studied but a number of recent studies suggest that phenelzine (an MAOI) and imipramine may reduce specific symptoms but have limited overall effect.

SOMATOFORM DISORDERS

Somatoform disorders represent a class of disorders that involve physical complaints that are without objective medical basis. Four major illnesses in this group are *somatization disorder, conversion disorder, psychogenic pain disorder,* and *hypochondriasis.* The prevalence rate of this group of disorders is approximately 0.1%, and women predominate. Psychogenic pain disorder has been reported to respond to antidepressant therapy. The other disorders have not been shown to be particularly responsive to psychopharmacologic therapy.

PERSONALITY DISORDERS

In DSM-III-R, personality disorder diagnoses are made under Axis II. Generally, these disorders have not been found to respond to psychopharmacologic treatment; however, medication may reduce certain symptoms. Three personality disorders are of particular note for this manual: borderline personality disorder, paranoid personality disorder, and antisocial personality disorder.

Borderline personality disorder, which has attracted great interest and study in recent years, is characterized by impulsivity; unstable and intense interpersonal relationships; inappropriate, intense anger; identity disturbances; affective instability; self-destructive physical acts; and a chronic sense of emptiness. This disorder (or variants thereof) may respond to lithium carbonate (emotionally unstable character), phenelzine (hysteroid dysphoria), low dosages of thioridazine, haloperidol, or thiothixene, and carbamazepine ("wrist slashers").

Paranoid personality disorder is characterized by pervasive unwarranted suspiciousness, hypersensitivity, and restricted affectivity. By definition, the paranoia is not due to schizophrenia or paranoid disorder. Although the somatic treatment of paranoid personality has not been well studied, trials of phenothiazines or lithium carbonate may prove useful in this disorder.

Antisocial personality disorder is characterized by chronic antisocial behavior, with onset before age 15. This disorder is far more common in men than in women. Six-month and lifetime prevalence rates for the disorder are approximately 0.8 and 2.5%, respectively.

PSYCHOACTIVE SUBSTANCE USE DISORDERS

Two major classes of substance abuse or dependence (alcohol and drugs) were emphasized in DSM-III. In DSM-III-R, criteria are provided for abuse and dependence of psychoactive substances in general. Abuse reflects pathologic use of a substance or impairment in social and occupational performance secondary to substance use. Dependence includes a psychological need for continuing a substance as well as abuse of, tolerance to, or characteristic symptoms on withdrawal from the particular substance.

The prevalence of substance use disorders is unfortunately high in the United States. Six-month and lifetime prevalence rates for alcohol dependence/abuse are approximately 5 and 13%, respectively. Alcohol abuse/dependence is five times more common in men than in women; drug abuse/dependence is somewhat less common, with 6-month and lifetime prevalence rates of 2 and 6%, respectively. Drug abuse/dependence is only slightly more common in men than in women.

In disorders involving substance use or abuse, pharmacologic treatment is generally aimed at ameliorating symptoms of withdrawal or at promoting abstinence either by producing physical discomfort in the face of intoxication (e.g., disulfiram for alcohol abuse) or by blocking drug-induced euphoria (e.g., methadone or naltrexone). When the substance has been abused in the context of another disorder (such as major depression), treatment of the underlying disorder is warranted (such as with a TCA).

"CHILDHOOD AND ADOLESCENT" DISORDERS

Two disorders that in DSM-III-R are subsumed under disorders of onset in childhood or adolescence deserve mention. *Bulimia,* characterized by intense eating binges, occurs in both adolescents and adults and has been thought by some investigators to be related to depression or affective disease. While there is some debate as to the nature of the possible relationship, it is clear that many bulimic patients respond to treatment with TCAs or MAOIs. Some bulimic patients also respond to behavior therapy. The other syndrome—*attention-deficit hyperactivity disorder*—is characterized by hyperactivity and poor attention span. Classically, it has its onset in childhood, but an adult form almost certainly exists (usually in patients who were hyperactive as children). The disorder responds well to stimulants and may also respond to TCAs and perhaps to MAOIs as well.

SUMMARY

Accurate diagnosis and classification provide clues for developing psychopharmacologic strategies. However, the clinician should not expect to find 1:1 correlations between the types of patients encountered in practice and the classic prototypes in the literature. This may prove particularly important when following a patient over many years. In such a case, a flexible approach needs to be developed, one that includes routine and regular reassessment of the patient's condition and the need for changes in medication. Table 2-2 illustrates the complex interdigitation of drug classes and

Table 2-2. Common and possible uses of classes of psychotropic medications

Antidepressant drugs	Major depressive disorders
	Agoraphobia with panic
	Panic
	Social phobias
	Bipolar disorders, depressed (with lithium)
	Generalized anxiety disorder
	Depression as a symptom in other primary disorders
	Psychogenic pain disorder
	Bulimia
Antipsychotic drugs	Schizophrenic disorder
	Schizophreniform disorder
	Schizoaffective disorder
	Bipolar disorder, manic phase
	Agitated organic disorders
	Borderline personality disorder
	Major depression with psychotic features
	? Treatment-resistant major depression
Antianxiety drugs	Generalized anxiety disorder
	Anxiety symptoms in other psychiatric disorders
	Akathisia
	Detoxification of alcohol dependence disorder
Stimulants	Adult attention-deficit disorder
	? Treatment-resistant depressive disorders
Lithium carbonate	Bipolar disorder
	Major depression (single episode or recurrent)
	Schizoaffective disorder
	? Impulse disorders
	? Cyclothymic disorder
Antiseizure drugs	Bipolar disorder
	Psychosis of temporal lobe epilepsy (TLE)
	? Major depression, treatment-resistant subtype with TLE features
	? Borderline personality disorder
	Schizoaffective disorder
	? Benzodiazepine withdrawal
Hypnotics	Sleep disturbance of mania, depression, anxiety, or other disorders

? indicates possible uses.

psychiatric disorders. These issues are discussed in more detail in the following chapters.

Bibliography

American Psychiatric Association: Diagnostic and Statistical Manual of Mental Disorders, 3rd Edition. Washington, DC, American Psychiatric Association, 1980

American Psychiatric Association: Diagnostic and Statistical Manual of Mental Disorders, 3rd Edition, Revised. Washington, DC, American Psychiatric Association, 1987

Bourdon KH, Boyd JH, Rae DS, et al: Gender differences in phobias: results of the ECA community survey. Journal of Anxiety Disorders 2:227–241, 1988

Boyd JH, Burke JD, Gruenberg E: Exclusion criteria of DSM-III: a study of co-occurrence of hierarchy-free syndromes. Arch Gen Psychiatry 41:983–989, 1984

Marks I, Lader M: Anxiety states (anxiety neurosis): a review. J Nerv Ment Dis 156:3–18, 1973

Myers JK, Weissman MM, Tischler GL, et al: Six-month prevalence of psychiatric disorders in three communities. Arch Gen Psychiatry 41:959–967, 1984

Pope HG, Lipinski JF: Diagnosis in schizophrenia and manic-depressive illness: a reassessment of the specificity of "schizophrenic" symptoms in the light of current research. Arch Gen Psychiatry 35:811–828, 1978

Regier DA, Boyd JH, Burke JD Jr, et al: One-month prevalence of mental disorders in the United States. Arch Gen Psychiatry 45:977–986, 1988

Regier DA, Narron WE, Rae DS: The epidemiology of anxiety disorders: the Epidemiologic Catchment Area (ECA) experience. J Psychiatr Res (in press)

Robins LN, Helzer JE, Weissman MM, et al: Lifetime prevalence of specific psychiatric disorders in three sites. Arch Gen Psychiatry 41:949–958, 1984

Schatzberg AF: Classification of affective disorders, in The Brain, Biochemistry, and Behavior (Proceedings of the Sixth Arnold O. Beckman Conference in Clinical Chemistry). Edited by Habig RL. Washington, DC, American Association for Clinical Chemistry, 1984, pp 29–46

Sheehan DV, Sheehan KH: The classification of anxiety and hysterical states, part I: historical review and empirical delineation. J Clin Psychopharmacol 2:235–244, 1982

Sheehan DV, Sheehan KH: The classification of anxiety and hysterical states, part II: towards a more heuristic classification. J Clin Psychopharmacol 2:386–393, 1982

Antidepressants

3

The class of drugs labeled as antidepressants has widened dramatically in the past 5 years with the introduction of several new compounds within this class. Classic antidepressants include the tricyclic antidepressants (TCAs) and related tetracyclics as well as the monoamine oxidase inhibitors (MAOIs). The newer agents (e.g., trazodone, bupropion, and fluoxetine) differ in structure from the classic medications and offer some advantages in terms of alternative biological actions and side-effect profiles. Overall, however, they are probably no more effective than previous pharmacologic agents. These newer medications may prove particularly useful for patients who cannot tolerate or have not responded to the more traditional agents. They are generally much less dangerous in overdose situations. For the clinician, learning to use them represents a great challenge, particularly when considering the task of trying to catch up with the ever-expanding and increasingly more complicated uses of traditional antidepressant medications.

Strengths and costs per 100 pills of individual antidepressants are found in the Appendix.

HISTORY

Classic antidepressants were originally discovered serendipitously. In the early 1950s, investigators noted that tuberculosis patients showed prolonged elevation of mood when treated with iproniazid, an MAOI thought to be an antituberculosis agent. This MAOI proved ineffective for tuberculosis, but its impact on mood led to some of the earliest double-blind studies in psychopharmacology, which demonstrated that MAOIs were effective antidepressant agents. The biologic and pharmacologic observations that MAOIs were antidepressants, and that monoamine oxidase degraded norepinephrine and serotonin, became cornerstones of the so-called biogenic amine theories of depression. Iproniazid, however, although available in Great Britain, was taken off the U.S. market some time ago because of fear that it caused hepatic necrosis. For many years the use of other MAOIs declined partly because of the introduction of TCAs, and partly because of the occurrence in patients of significant hypertensive crises.

TCAs were also discovered serendipitously. The first reports on TCA efficacy in depression came from Professor Kuhn in Switzerland, who astutely noted that a three-ringed compound, imipramine, which was being investigated as a treatment for schizophrenia, appeared to elevate mood even though it did not relieve psychosis. The drug was similar in structure to the phenothiazines but a simple substitution of nitrogen for sulfur in the central ring appeared to confer unique psychopharmacologic antidepressant properties.

Two of the newer antidepressants with a four-ringed structure, maprotiline and amoxapine, share similar biochemical effects with the more traditional TCAs. This is not unexpected, since many antidepressant compounds were developed based on their having similar activity in certain animal models to those of prototypic TCAs, leading some to call them "me too" drugs. However, there are both subtle and pronounced differences between many of the so-called me too drugs. More recently, three new compounds—trazodone, fluoxetine, and bupropion—with rather unique biological properties have been introduced to the U.S. market. These, along with a host of investigational drugs developed using alternative animal screening, truly represent the second generation of antidepressant drugs.

TRICYCLIC ANTIDEPRESSANTS AND RELATED COMPOUNDS

Indications

The principal "Food and Drug Administration (FDA)-approved for marketing" indication for TCAs and related compounds is the treatment of depression—both endogenous and nonendogenous. Other "approved for marketing" indications include anxiety (doxepin) and childhood enuresis (imipramine as an adjunctive treatment). "Nonapproved" but common uses include insomnia (particularly amitriptyline and doxepin), headache (most commonly amitriptyline, imipramine, and doxepin), agoraphobia with panic attacks (imipramine particularly), chronic pain syndromes (doxepin and maprotiline most frequently), and bulimia (imipramine and desipramine). More recently, imipramine has been reported effective in generalized anxiety disorder, and trimipramine and doxepin may be effective in treating peptic ulcers. The recently released TCA clomipramine has potent anti–obsessive-compulsive effects, as probably do the new, pure serotonin reuptake blockers (e.g., fluoxetine). Obviously, these drugs exert rather wide pharmacologic effects, which account for their potentially broad range of actions. (For further discussion of the use of TCAs in anxiety disorders, see the section on antidepressants in Chapter 6.)

There are currently eight tricyclic and two tetracyclic antidepressants on the U.S. market. One tricyclic, clomipramine, is approved for the treatment of obsessive-compulsive disorder but not for depression. It is used worldwide, however, as a major antidepressant. Trade and generic names of the tricyclic and tetracyclic antidepressants are listed in Table 3-1. The original patents have expired on several of them, for which generic preparations are now available. In the United States, generic compounds have not been without controversy. Although they offer a savings for the consumer, some clinicians question their pharmacologic equivalence. One difficulty stems from the FDA definition of bioequivalence, which has relied heavily on the demonstration that an identical dosage of a generic preparation produces blood levels within a specified range 20–30% above and below those produced by the original compound. Even with approved generics, some studies have suggested that they are not truly equivalent to standard brands. Moreover, the regulations have not required that pharmaceutical companies prove that their generics enjoy equivalence in clinical or biological potency. This area needs close scrutiny by both clinicians and investigators. At the time of writing, FDA regulations for generic preparations were being revised.

Structures

The chemical structures of TCAs and related compounds are remarkably similar (Figure 3-1). Desipramine and nortriptyline are demethylated metabolites of imipramine and amitriptyline, respectively. Amoxapine is a derivative of the antipsychotic loxapine and has an additional fourth ring off a side chain. Maprotiline is a four-ring compound, the fourth ring arising perpendicular to the traditional three rings. Its side chain is identical to that of desipramine.

Table 3-1. Tricyclic and tetracyclic antidepressants

Generic name	Brand names	Tablets and capsules	Oral concentrate	Parenteral	Therapeutic dosage range (mg/day)*
Tricyclics					
amitriptyline†	Elavil, Endep	Tablet: 10, 25, 50, 75, 100, 150 mg	None	10 mg/ml in 10-ml vials	150–300
clomipramine	Anafranil	Capsule: 25, 50, 75 mg	None	None	100–250
desipramine†	Norpramin Pertofrane	Tablet: 10, 25, 50, 75, 100, 150 mg	None	None	150–300
doxepin†	Sinequan Adapin	Capsule: 25, 50 mg Capsule: 10, 25, 50, 75, 100, 150 mg	10 mg/ml in 120-ml bottles	None	150–300
imipramine†	Tofranil Janimine Sk-Pramine	Tablet: 10, 25, 50 mg	None	25 mg in 2-ml vials	150–300
imipramine pamoate	Tofranil PM (sustained release)	Capsule: 75, 100, 125, 150 mg‡	None	25 mg in 2-ml vials	150–300
nortriptyline	Pamelor Aventyl	Capsule: 10, 25, 50, 75 mg	10 mg/5 ml in 16-oz bottles	None	50–150
protriptyline	Vivactil	Tablet: 5, 10 mg	None	None	15–60
trimipramine†	Surmontil	Capsule: 25, 50, 100 mg	None	None	150–300
Tetracyclics					
amoxapine	Asendin	Tablet: 25, 50, 100, 150 mg	None	None	150–450
maprotiline†	Ludiomil	Tablet: 25, 50, 75 mg	None	None	150–200

* Dosage ranges are approximate. Many patients will respond at relatively low dosages (even below ranges given above); others may require higher dosages.
† Available in generic form.
‡ Imipramine 100-mg and 125-mg capsules contain tartrazine.

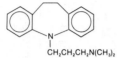

Imipramine

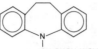

Trimipramine

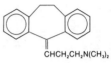

Amitriptyline

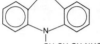

Desipramine

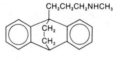

Doxepin

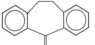

Nortriptyline

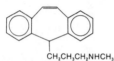

Protriptyline

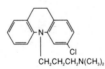

Maprotiline

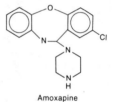

Amoxapine

Clomipramine hydrochloride

Figure 3-1. Chemical structures of tricyclic and related antidepressants.

Biochemical Effects

The biochemical effects of these tricyclic and tetracyclic antidepressants are quite similar. Initially, particular emphasis was placed on their relative effects in blocking the reuptake of norepinephrine or serotonin. These differences came to underlie various theories on the biology of depression—

particularly the low norepinephrine versus low serotonin hypotheses. In recent years, theories have become more complex as the pharmacologic effects of these drugs have been shown to go beyond their mere immediate reuptake blocking effects to include later secondary effects on pre- and postsynaptic receptors, as well as on other neurotransmitter systems. The latter effects may account for differences among the various drugs in both their range of efficacy and their side effects. At one time, the relative norepinephrine versus serotonin reuptake blocking effects were used to explain the relative sedative (serotonin) versus activating (norepinephrine) properties of these drugs. More recently, sedation, which early on was ascribed to serotonergic and anticholinergic effects, has in part been ascribed to tricyclics' antihistamine (H_1 receptor) actions. Some investigators have argued that weight gain could also be due to H_1 receptor blocking effects. Anticholinergic effects include dry mouth, constipation, urinary hesitance, blurred vision, and confusion. The H_2 receptor blocking effects may play a role in these drugs, promoting healing of peptic ulcers.

The relative norepinephrine versus serotonin (5-HT) reuptake blocking effects of the non-MAOI antidepressants are summarized in Table 3-2. Their relative effects on acetylcholine, H_1, H_2, alpha$_1$, 5-HT$_1$, and 5-HT$_2$ receptors are summarized in Table 3-3. These potencies represent best estimates based on receptor-binding and clinical studies. Note that the TCAs currently available in the United States are relatively weak serotonin reuptake blockers. Clomipramine is the one exception to this rule. Indeed, in some in vivo models, TCAs—other than clomipramine—are devoid of serotonin blocking effects, as is trazodone. Moreover, recent research points to some of the antidepressants as having serotonin receptor blocking effects, suggesting that some are serotonin antagonists. Taken together, laboratory data suggest that the tricyclics—other than clomipramine (see Chapter 6)—are weak serotonergic agents. In contrast, fluoxetine and fluvoxamine

Table 3-2. Norepinephrine (NE) and serotonin (5-HT) uptake blockage effects of antidepressants

	NE	5-HT
amitriptyline	+	+ +
desipramine	+ + +	+
doxepin	+	+
imipramine	+	+ +
nortriptyline	+ +	+
protriptyline	+ + +	+
trimipramine	0	0
amoxapine	+ +	+
maprotiline	+ +	0
trazodone •	0	+
fluoxetine	0	+ + +
fluvoxamine	0	+ + +
clomipramine	+ +	+ + +
bupropion	0	0

Note. Approximations of relative activity from in vivo, in vitro, and clinical studies. Data on clomipramine include results on desmethylclomipramine on active metabolite with pronounced effects on NE systems. In certain in vivo models, the tricyclic antidepressants (other than clomipramine) and trazodone have been reported to *not* block 5-HT uptake. 0 = no effect. + + + = marked effect.

are relatively pure serotonin reuptake blockers with little in the way of antagonist effects. Thus, these drugs do offer an alternative for the clinician (see below). The tricyclic and tetracyclic antidepressants are virtually devoid of dopamine reuptake blocking effects. Of available antidepressants, only bupropion has dopamine reuptake blocking effects, albeit somewhat weak. Variations in biological effects help in drug selection, both in terms of clinical efficacy and side effects. Table 3-4 indicates the types of side effects seen with tricyclic and tetracyclic compounds.

Dosage Regimens

Having evaluated a depressed patient, the clinician must determine whether TCAs appear to be an appropriate treat-

Table 3-3. Relative receptor blocking effects of antidepressants

	ACh	α_1	H_1	5-HT$_1$	5-HT$_2$
amitriptyline	+ + +	+ + +	+ +	±	+
desipramine	+	+	+	0	±
doxepin	+ +	+ + +	+ + +	±	+
imipramine	+ +	+	+	0	+
nortriptyline	+	+	+	±	+
protriptyline	+ + +	+	+	0	+
trimipramine	+ +	+ +	+ + +	0	+
amoxapine	+	+ +	+	±	+ + +
maprotiline	+	+	+ +	0	±
trazodone	0	+ +	±	+	+ +
fluoxetine	0	0	0	0	±
fluvoxamine	0	0	0	0	0
clomipramine	+	+ +	+	0	+
bupropion	0	0	0	0	0

Note. Data presented are approximations of relative activity from in vivo, in vitro, and clinical studies. Receptors: ACh = muscarinic acetylcholine. α_1 = alpha$_1$-adrenergic. H_1 = histamine 1. 5-HT$_1$ = serotonin 1. 5-HT$_2$ = serotonin 2. 0 = no effect. + + + = marked effect.

ment. In our first edition of this manual, we subscribed to the approach of using a TCA first in the treatment of endogenous or major depression. Currently, as we are writing this second edition, we are becoming more impressed with the serotonin reuptake blocker fluoxetine as a potential first-order medication, particularly in outpatients in whom efficacy has been clearly demonstrated in double-blind studies (see below).

Which TCA to use is somewhat a matter of personal preference. There is really considerable overlap among these various drugs, although some are a bit more stimulating (desipramine and protriptyline) and others are more sedating (amitriptyline and doxepin). One of us (A.F.S.) tends to start with imipramine, the oldest of these drugs; J.O.C. tends to use imipramine when more sedation is required and desipramine where sedation is potentially a problem. Neither of us

Table 3-4. Common or troublesome side effects of tricyclic and tetracyclic drugs

---

● **Anticholinergic**
Dry mouth and nasal passages, constipation, urinary hesitance, esophageal reflux

● **Autonomic**
Orthostatic hypotension, palpitations, intracardiac conduction slowing, increased sweating, increased blood pressure, tremor

● **Allergic**
Skin rashes (particularly with maprotiline)

● **Central Nervous System**
Stimulation, sedation, delirium, myoclonic twitches (generally at high dosages), nausea, speech blockage, seizures (particularly with high dosages of maprotiline), and extrapyramidal symptoms (amoxapine)

● **Other**
Weight gain and impotence

---

employs amitriptyline as a first-choice treatment. The drug is obviously effective but often too sedating, as indicated by its wide use as both an antidepressant and a sedative-hypnotic. We have found that many patients cannot tolerate amitriptyline's marked anticholinergic side effects, which include a sense of spaciness that can occur more commonly with this drug, as well as marked dry mouth, constipation, etc.

With any of these drugs the clinician is best advised to start with a relatively low dose, which can then be increased slowly. For imipramine the starting doses and regimens vary. One common imipramine regimen is to prescribe 75 mg/day during week 1, and to increase weekly, as needed, to 150 mg/day during week 2, 225 mg/day during week 3, and 300 mg/day during week 4. Another approach is to start at 50 mg/day, increasing the dose, as tolerated, by 25 mg/day to 150 mg/day and after some 2 weeks increasing from 150 mg at a rate of 50 mg every 3 days to 300 mg/day. (Similar dosage regimens are recommended for other uses of the drug—panic, pain, etc.) For some patients, particularly the elderly, it seems reasonable to begin at 25 mg on day 1 and increase to 50 mg on day 2, allowing the patient to become acclimated to a single small dose. We also advise a more conservative schedule of increases, remaining at 50 mg/day for 1 week and thereafter increasing the dosage at a rate of 25 mg every 2 days to 150 mg/day. After 7 days on 150 mg/day, the dosage can be increased further as tolerated. The elderly present a somewhat unique problem (see Chapter 12). The not uncommon medical problems of the elderly and their relatively slow drug metabolism usually dictate conservative management; however, clinicians must be careful since some elderly patients are not slow metabolizers but instead require reasonably high dosages and run the risk of being undertreated. The degree of side effects can be a useful barometer as to the ability to tolerate a given dosage, and plasma levels may aid in prescribing optimal doses (see below sections "Tricyclic Blood Levels" and "Side Effects").

For doxepin, amitriptyline, and trimipramine, dosage ranges similar to those for imipramine are recommended both in younger and older patients. We have recently been impressed with trimipramine's relatively low side effect profile in the elderly and with its rapid effects on promoting sleep. Nortriptyline and protriptyline are prescribed in rather different ways. In younger patients, protriptyline is generally started at 15 mg (5 mg tid) in week 1 with increases of 5–10 mg/week to a maximum of 60 mg/day. (In the elderly, begin at 10 mg/day.) Nortriptyline, which is the only TCA to clearly have a so-called therapeutic window, can be ineffective if the patient attains either too low or too high plasma levels. The therapeutic dosage range for nortriptyline in adults is 50–150 mg/day. We recommend starting at 50 mg/day and increasing at a rate of 50 mg/week. (In the elderly, begin at 25 mg/day and increase to 50 mg/day after 3 or 4 days.) After 3 weeks, a decrease in dosage may actually be helpful, a state of affairs rather different from the other TCAs (see below section "Tricyclic Blood Levels"). Amoxapine's starting dose in healthy adults is 150 mg/day with a maximum daily dose of 400 mg/day. Maprotiline's starting and maximum dosages are 75 and 225 mg/day, respectively. To avoid seizures, the starting dose of maprotiline should be maintained for 2 weeks, and after 6 weeks of treatment, the dosage should be reduced to a maximum of 175 mg/day.

The response to TCAs is slower than one would hope. Traditionally, the rule of thumb has been that it takes 2 weeks for patients to begin to respond and that patients who are going to respond will begin to show some positive effects by 4 weeks. (One notable exception is amoxapine, which may work in as little as 4 days and enjoys a claim for more rapid onset.) Quitkin et al. (1984) reviewed a large series of depressed patients who were treated with traditional TCAs and concluded that relatively few patients demonstrate significant improvement after only 2 weeks of therapy and many require as long as 6 weeks to respond. Our group has reported that slow and rapid responders to maprotiline could be identified biologically by their pretreatment urinary levels of 3-methoxy-4-hydroxyphenylglycol (MHPG), which is indicative of norepinephrine function. Patients with low MHPG levels demonstrate rapid responses (in less than 14 days), and those with very high MHPG levels need 4–6 weeks of treatment.

What should the clinician do if after 6 weeks the patient has either demonstrated a partial response or has not responded at all? First, the clinician should consider increasing the dosage (unless the maximum maprotiline dose has been attained), since some patients are rapid—and not slow—drug metabolizers. Here, too, plasma levels can be a guide for increasing the dosage and determining how high to go (see below section "Tricyclic Blood Levels"). For other patients, the addition of lithium carbonate or Cytomel (T_3) can bring out a clinical response (see Chapter 9). If these additions do not produce a response, the clinician is faced with the option of either changing the drug or moving on to electroconvulsive therapy.

For many years and still today in many centers, clinicians will choose to switch from one TCA to another. Increasingly, we have become dissatisfied with this approach. Our experience has been that patients who have tolerated, but have not responded to, an adequate trial on one TCA will rarely respond to an adequate trial of a second. All too often we have seen patients who have had multiple unsuccessful TCA trials. We recommend switching to another class of treatment sooner than was previously common.

Another recent strategy has been to add fluoxetine to the TCA. The combination in lower animals produced pronounced pharmacological downregulation of postsynaptic receptors, suggesting the combination should be potent in humans. One important caveat must be raised. Fluoxetine will increase TCA plasma levels as much as threefold; clinicians should thus reduce the TCA gradually to relatively low doses (less than 50 mg nortriptyline) before adding fluoxetine (see Chapter 9).

If the patient responds, how long should he or she stay on the drug? Here, too, clinical thinking has changed. Early practice was to keep patients on the drug for a few months. Currently, practice has moved to longer-term maintenance treatment of at least 6–12 months to prevent early relapse. In a recent major National Institute of Mental Health (NIMH) collaborative study (Prien et al. 1984), imipramine was generally more effective than placebo or lithium in preventing relapse of major depression over a 2-year maintenance period. In contrast to this study, two earlier major studies, here and in the United Kingdom, found lithium to be as effective as the TCA in preventing relapses in unipolar depressed patients. In the study by Prien et al. (1984), the overall relapse rate in the unipolar group was relatively high (overall relapse rate, 64%; imipramine group, 49%), and the authors even argued for the need to develop newer, alternative strategies, perhaps with drugs other than TCAs. (For further discussion of maintenance therapy in affective disorders, see Chapter 4.)

In the first edition of this manual, we indicated that after being maintained for some 3–4 months on the doses at which they responded, many patients can be maintained at lower doses (one-half to three-quarters that of the original dose) for the remaining months. However, a recent report indicates that this may not be the case. Currently, we recommend maintaining patients at their therapeutic dosage levels unless pronounced side effects are present. If the patient begins to relapse on the same dose to which he or she had previously responded, the addition of 25 μg/day of Cytomel will often bring about a renewed response (see Chapter 9). Another option is to recheck the plasma level; if it is not high, the dosage can be increased to bring the plasma level into the so-called therapeutic range (see below). This area is confusing for the clinician and the patient, who naturally wonder whether the drug's effect has worn off or a natural recurrence has taken place.

Fortunately, maintenance on tricyclics or other antidepressants is generally not associated with particular major long-term side effects in contrast to those seen with lithium (thyroid goiter) or antipsychotics (tardive dyskinesia). (Again, maprotiline's maintenance dosage should not exceed 175 mg/day.) However, as described below, long-term use of the MAOIs does pose a cumulative, increased risk for acute hypertensive crises occurring (see below) should an unsuspecting patient ingest certain foodstuffs or other medications. Also, alprazolam used for prolonged periods can possibly result in dependence (see Chapter 6).

When discontinuing or tapering tricyclics, it is most prudent to do so at a maximum rate of 25–50 mg every 2–3 days. Many patients will demonstrate symptoms of cholinergic rebound if the TCA is discontinued too abruptly. These include nausea, queasy stomach, cramping, sweating, headache, neck pain, vomiting, etc. We have observed several patients who experienced intense gastrointestinal symptoms on TCA withdrawal. For these patients, propantheline bromide (15 mg tid prn) has been extremely helpful. Moreover, we reported that some patients will demonstrate "rebound" hypomania or mania with sudden cessation of TCAs, an observation confirmed by others.

When the issue of rebound symptoms versus a medical illness or recurrence of psychiatric symptoms is in doubt, a single dose of the discontinued drug will often relieve the symptoms rapidly, confirming the diagnosis of a withdrawal syndrome. There is one report in which withdrawal mania responded to reinstitution of desipramine therapy (Nelson et al. 1983).

Tricyclic Blood Levels

In past decades, considerable attention has been paid to the use of drug blood levels to monitor treatment with various psychotropic agents. Currently, blood levels are most commonly used in patients treated with TCAs, neuroleptics, lithium carbonate, and anticonvulsants. Blood levels for benzodiazepines are neither widely available nor commonly used. Drug concentrations are determined primarily in serum (e.g., for lithium carbonate and anticonvulsants) or plasma (e.g., for TCAs). In addition to measuring the concentration of neuroleptics in blood, some laboratories also measure the relative binding to dopamine receptors (so-called radioreceptor assays).

Generally, blood levels are determined in blood drawn 8–12 hours after the patient's last dose in an effort to avoid "false" peaks in blood levels that would occur if blood was drawn immediately after a patient had taken the medication. Also, plasma levels are most accurate when drawn after the patient has achieved "steady state"—the point at which a specific dose of drug given over a several-day period produces a consistent blood level. For TCAs this is approximately 5–7 days.

Plasma levels can be particularly useful barometers of drug metabolism. There is approximately a 30-fold difference among human subjects in plasma levels of TCAs produced by a single fixed milligram per kilogram dose of a drug, reflecting the degree to which the slowest and fastest metabolizers differ in drug absorption and metabolism. Obviously, slow metabolizers (such as the elderly) are at a higher risk for becoming toxic; fast metabolizers may have difficulty building drug levels. Most patients, however, fall in the middle range of the normal bell-shaped curve distribution.

For TCAs, the clearest use is in patients with endogenous depression. There is little or no relationship between TCA level and clinical response in patients with nonendogenous depression or those with dysthymia. Two types of relationships between TCA levels and clinical response in endogenously depressed patients have been described in the literature. Glassman et al. (1977) have reported a sigmoidal relationship between response and imipramine plus desipramine levels; clinical response increases with plasma level up to approximately 250 ng/ml and then levels off thereafter (Figure 3-2). Glassman has reported rates of response of 30%, 67%, and 93%, for patients with plasma levels in the following ranges: less than 150, 150–225, and greater than 225 ng/ml. For nortriptyline, a curvilinear relationship has been described, as indicated in Figure 3-3. Response increases with plasma level and then plateaus in the range of approximately 50–150 ng/ml with a decrease in response at plasma levels greater than 150 ng/ml. The critical 50–150 ng/ml range has been called the therapeutic window. Nonresponding patients with plasma levels of approximately 150 ng/ml may respond to a lowering of dosage and plasma level into the window. The decreased responsivity above the window is not due to side effects. Therapeutic windows have at times been described

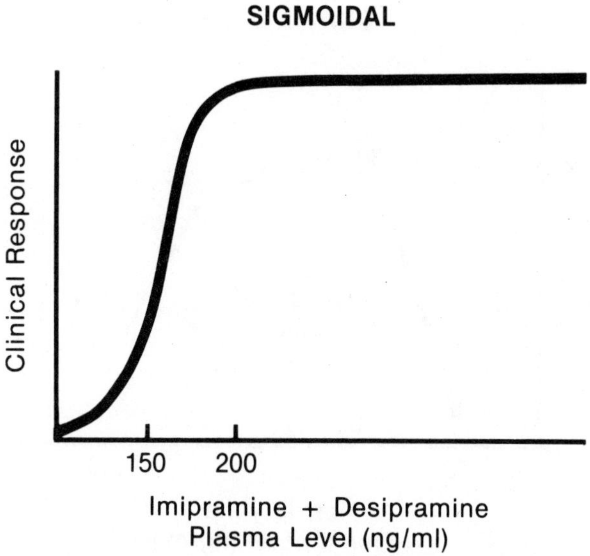

SIGMOIDAL

Clinical Response

150   200

Imipramine + Desipramine
Plasma Level (ng/ml)

Figure 3-2. Sigmoidal relationship between clinical response and imipramine plus desipramine plasma levels.

for other drugs, but these are not as clear as with nortriptyline. Approximate therapeutic plasma levels are summarized in Table 3-5.

A number of medications may increase or decrease plasma levels—generally by interfering with or augmenting liver microsomal enzyme activity. For example, nicotine, barbiturates (including Fiorinal), chloral hydrate, phenytoin, and carbamazepine induce breakdown of TCAs, and clinicians should keep this in mind when prescribing TCAs to patients who are taking the above compounds. In contrast, antipsychotics (particularly phenothiazines), methylphenidate, disulfiram, and fenfluramine will increase plasma levels by slowing drug metabolism in the liver. Recently, we have observed that fluoxetine may also substantially increase TCA blood levels.

CURVILINEAR

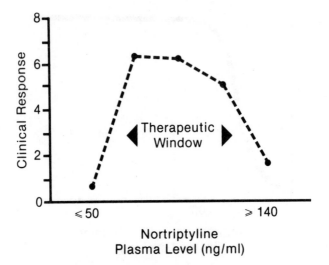

Figure 3-3. Curvilinear relationship between clinical response and nortriptyline plasma levels.

Conversely, TCAs increase phenothiazine plasma levels as well. Benzodiazepines and antiparkinsonian medications have little or no effect on TCA levels, although there is one report that alprazolam will increase imipramine blood levels.

A number of issues arise when one considers plasma level data. For one, studies generally use fixed milligram per kilogram dosing such that it is possible that a patient with a given TCA plasma level (e.g., 250 ng/ml) on a given dose (e.g., 300 mg/day of imipramine) might well have responded to a lower dosage and at a lower plasma level. In a sense, then, plasma levels can be viewed as barometers of adequacy of treatment. Patients who are not responding to a 4- to 6-week trial of imipramine but who have attained a plasma level of 150 ng/ml or less may respond to an increase in dosage and plasma level to greater than 200 ng/ml. On the other hand, another patient who is responding at exactly the

Table 3-5. Approximate therapeutic plasma level ranges for tricyclic and tetracyclic drugs

Drug	Blood level (ng/ml)
amitriptyline	100–250*
desipramine	150–300
doxepin	120–250*
imipramine	150–300*
nortriptyline†	50–150
protriptyline	75–250
trimipramine	Unknown
amoxapine	Unknown
maprotiline	150–250

* Total concentration of drug and demethylated metabolite.
† Has a clear therapeutic window.

same dosage and plasma level does not need to have the dosage or plasma level increased even if it is below the therapeutic range. Some investigators have advocated determining the plasma level for any patient who is responding to a TCA so as to record *that patient's* therapeutic plasma level on that drug. This could prove important if the patient has a later recurrence and requires retreatment.

Sometimes a routine check of a TCA blood level in a patient who is clinically much improved and has only minor side effects will reveal a plasma level of greater than 400 ng/ml, and the patient will relapse when the dose is decreased to bring down the plasma level. This result suggests that, for that particular patient, a very high plasma level was necessary for improvement. Indeed, there was a prospective report that some patients require very high dosages and blood levels to respond, although there is an inherent risk in this approach.

So far, only amitriptyline shows clear toxicity related to plasma levels around 500 ng/ml. Obviously, clinical judgment is necessary. ECG is useful in patients who do well only on very high plasma levels to ensure that cardiac conduction is not seriously affected—i.e., to ensure against intracardiac conduction slowing.

Another practical problem has revolved around the variation among laboratories in their TCA assays. This is of
major importance since clinicians may be unable to interpret
a given value in their laboratories. A major national effort
has been underway to cross-validate laboratories, and this
problem appears to be resolving. Physicians should check
with their laboratories as to whether quality control methods
are routinely employed. At any rate, plasma levels can provide
useful clinical information if the clinician keeps these issues
in mind.

Side Effects

A review of PDR package insert information on each of the
TCAs and related agents indicates their myriad side effects.
These can be grouped broadly by categories: anticholinergic,
autonomic, allergic, etc. (Table 3-4). This organization is
somewhat artificial, since a single side effect (e.g., sedation)
may actually be due to any number of distinct neurochemical
effects (e.g., histamine blockade, increased serotonin availability, and others, or combinations thereof). In addition, some
side effects may reflect drug action in either the brain or the
periphery or in both (e.g., orthostatic hypotension).

How can clinicians help in the management of side effects?
In some patients, particularly those with complicating medical
illnesses, side reactions may not be entirely controllable or
manageable. There are, however, some things that can be
done, particularly for less severe reactions in medically healthy
patients.

One very important issue is attitude. Not uncommonly,
some psychiatrists have rather negative views about medication, and these can be communicated indirectly or overtly
to the patient, particularly if the impetus to try medications
has arisen from the patient and not the physician. In our
experience, this attitude can be troubling to the patient, who
must rely on the physician's belief in the importance of

medication trials and in being able to deal with the side effects. It is thus imperative for clinicians to develop well-reasoned and balanced views about prescribing drugs.

A general principle of drug prescribing is that some side effects can be managed by reducing the dosage or can be avoided by increasing it slowly. In our experience this is particularly true for the early emergence of "spaciness," depersonalization, confusion, orthostatic hypotension, or marked sedation. If these reactions persist in the presence of more moderate dose escalation, a switch to another TCA or another class of drug may be necessary. In dealing with anticholinergic side effects or sedation, switching to desipramine seems reasonable. For patients who develop orthostatic hypotension, nortriptyline is often a useful alternative, since it tends to produce orthostatic changes at plasma levels above the so-called therapeutic window. Thus it is more easily tolerated than imipramine, whose orthostatic effects are often produced at low plasma levels (see preceding section "Tricyclic Blood Levels"). Nortriptyline has been used successfully in several studies on poststroke depression.

Peripheral anticholinergic side effects have also been reported to be ameliorated by administering bethanechol, a procholinergic drug, in doses of 25–50 mg given three or four times daily. Generally this is continued for as long as the patient remains on TCAs. This drug can be particularly helpful to patients with urinary hesitancy. In cases of anticholinergic deliria, physostigmine (a centrally acting procholinergic agent) may be administered either intravenously or intramuscularly to clarify the diagnosis. (For specific information regarding the use of physostigmine, see Chapter 9.)

Blurred vision as a result of TCAs can be treated with 4% pilocarpine drops or with oral bethanechol. Patients otherwise doing well on maintenance TCA treatment and therefore likely to be on the drug for some time may require a change in their eyeglass prescription to correct the blurring of vision.

For severe dry mouth, a 1% pilocarpine solution can be created by mixing the 4% solution available as eyedrops with three parts water. This solution can be swished around the mouth for a few minutes, 30 minutes to an hour before the increase in salivation is expected. For example, patients may use this mouthwash before having to give a lecture. Bethanechol in 5- or 10-mg tablets may be administered sublingually for a similar effect.

An important, possibly antihistaminic side effect of TCAs is weight gain—particularly seen with amitriptyline and doxepin—which can be difficult to control pharmacologically. Often, patients who demonstrate this side effect on one TCA will continue to gain weight when switched to another related drug. In some patients, switching to trazodone, bupropion, or fluoxetine may be the only way to maintain an antidepressant effect and promote weight reduction (see sections below), since MAOIs will also cause weight gain. Unfortunately, there are patients who still continue to gain weight while receiving the drug to which they are showing an antidepressant response. In such cases, support and advice regarding dieting may be the only recourse.

Two of the newer compounds—maprotiline and amoxapine—have been reported to produce troublesome side effects—seizures and extrapyramidal symptoms—that have been less frequently reported with the standard TCAs. Induced seizures have been reported in a number of single case reports using maprotiline. Recently, our group reported a series of 11 seizure patients at one hospital and a study of all U.S. maprotiline-related seizures. In our series, prolonged treatment (longer than 6 weeks) at high dosages (225–400 mg/day) appeared to be a major factor. This was confirmed in the U.S. survey. In addition, rapid dose escalation—reaching 150 mg/day within 7 days—was a major factor in the general survey. When these two factors were eliminated, the risk of seizures appeared to approximate that associated with classic antidepressants (approximately 0.2%). The manufacturer of maprotiline has altered its dosage guidelines, recommending beginning treatment at 75 mg/day for 2 weeks, a maximum dose of 225 mg/day for up to 6 weeks, and maintenance at 200 mg/day or below. The previous dosage schedule had been similar to that of imipramine.

Amoxapine has been reported to produce a number of side effects associated with dopamine receptor blockade—e.g., galactorrhea, akathisia, and other extrapyramidal symptoms—and even a few cases of dyskinesia, similar to those more commonly found with the neuroleptic loxapine. Amoxapine is metabolized generally to a 7-OH metabolite. In some individuals, alternate hydroxylation at the 8 position results in the accumulation of a neuroleptic metabolite. Generally speaking, we recommend tapering or stopping medications if these symptoms occur (see the preceding section "Tricyclic Blood Levels").

MONOAMINE OXIDASE INHIBITORS

The primary PDR clinical indication for MAOIs is for depression that is refractory to tricyclic therapy. Phenelzine enjoys an indication for anxious depression. Although the British have emphasized frequently that the MAOIs are not particularly helpful in endogenous depression, the American experience, including our own, has been entirely different. These drugs have been lifesavers for many endogenously depressed patients, particularly those who have failed to respond to TCAs.

Why the discrepancy? For one, there is little doubt that MAOIs are effective in patients with panic attacks or with anxious or atypical depression. However, their effectiveness in endogenous depression may require the prescription of considerably higher dosages than the early British trials, which used relatively low dosages. Another difficulty with determining ranges of efficacy revolves around the occurrence of pronounced obsessionality, agitation, and anxiety in many endogenously depressed patients who may in early studies have been misdiagnosed as atypically depressed.

In recent years, investigators at Columbia University have attempted to define an atypical depressive syndrome that preferentially responds to phenelzine. Their data suggest that atypical depressive patients respond better to phenelzine than imipramine.

The first-generation MAOIs—isocarboxazid, phenelzine, and tranylcypromine—have few direct effects on reuptake or receptor blockade. Instead, they inhibit monoamine oxidase (MAO) in various organs, exerting greater effects on MAO A—for which norepinephrine and serotonin are primary substrates—than on MAO B, which acts primarily on other amines, e.g., phenylethylamine. Also, MAO B is found in the gut and is responsible for degrading various amines that can act as false neurotransmitters and produce hypertensive crises (see below). Isocarboxazide, phenelzine, and tranylcypromine are so-called irreversible inhibitors. When the enzyme is inhibited by these agents, protein regeneration is required before MAO enzymatic activity is restored. This requires considerable time, up to 2 weeks. Thus, untoward side effects due to ingestion of certain foodstuffs are not reversed by merely stopping the drug, and cessation of MAOIs must be coupled with continuation of a special diet for some 2 weeks after stopping. Selegiline (deprenyl), a new MAO-reversible inhibitor used in parkinsonian patients, exerts its effects on MAO A and is generally thought to have very low risk for producing hypertensive crises. However, at the low dosages used in parkinsonian patients, this drug is a weak antidepressant, and recent data from Sunderland and colleagues (1989) suggest that at higher antidepressant dosages, the drug affects both MAO A and B and thus does not protect against hypertensive crises. More information on selegiline is provided in a separate subsection of this chapter.

There are two structural classes of MAOIs: the hydrazines—isocarboxazid and phenelzine—and the nonhydra-

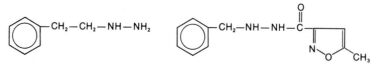

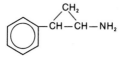

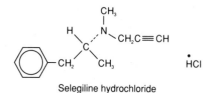

Figure 3-4. Chemical structures of monoamine oxidase inhibitors.

zine—tranylcypromine and selegiline (see Figure 3-4 and Table 3-6).

Dosages

The traditional therapeutic dosage ranges of these three MAOIs are isocarboxazid, 20–30 mg/day; phenelzine, 45–90 mg/day; and tranylcypromine, 30–60 mg/day. Most patients will require treatment at the higher end of the dosage range. For example, 90 mg/day of phenelzine is commonly required in a patient with severe depressive illness.

A patient treated with phenelzine should be started at 30 mg/day and increased to 45 mg/day after 3 days. Thereafter, the dosage can be increased at a rate of 15 mg/week to 90 mg/day. We have seen patients who require as much as 120 mg/day; however, many patients cannot tolerate the orthostatic side effects of these drugs. Some investigators have recommended a 1 mg/kg per day dose of the drug as a guideline for adequacy of treatment.

For tranylcypromine, a starting dose of 20 mg/day for 3 days seems reasonable. This can then be increased to 30 mg/day for 1 week with 10 mg/day increases to 50–60 mg/day.

Table 3-6. Monoamine oxidase inhibitors (MAOIs) and other available drugs

Generic name	Brand name	Tablets	Oral concentrate	Parenteral	Usual therapeutic dosage (mg/day)*
MAOIs					
isocarboxazid	Marplan	10 mg	None	None	30–50
phenelzine	Nardil	15 mg	None	None	45–90
selegiline	Eldepryl	5 mg	None	None	20–50
tranylcypromine	Parnate	10 mg	None	None	30–50
Other					
bupropion	Wellbutrin	75, 100 mg	None	None	200–450
fluoxetine	Prozac	Capsules: 20 mg	None	None	20–60
trazodone	Desyrel, Generic	50, 100, 150 mg†	None	None	150–300

* Dosage ranges are approximate. Many patients will respond at relatively low dosages (even below ranges given above); others may require higher dosages.
† Trazodone is also available in 100- and 300-mg divided-dose forms.

The current recommended maximum dose of the drug is 40 mg/day. One investigator, Dr. Jay Amsterdam, has reported that extremely high doses of the drug (110–130 mg/day) may help even the most refractory of depressed patients. There is some thought that at such high doses the drug is exerting alternative, additional effects, possibly acting as a reuptake blocker (Amsterdam and Berwish 1989). Isocarboxazid, which is less commonly prescribed than the others, should be titrated at a rate similar to the usual schedule for tranylcypromine. Its recommended maximum daily dosage is 30 mg/day, and the manufacturer indicates it can be started at that dose as well. Higher doses, up to 50 mg/day, have been required for many patients. Once a patient has responded, the medication should be maintained for a length of time similar to that recommended for the tricyclics.

Side Effects

Common side effects of MAOIs are listed in Table 3-7. Since MAOIs are not purported to block acetylcholine receptors, they produce less in the way of dry mouth, blurred vision, constipation, and urinary hesitancy. However, we have seen patients who have developed urinary hesitancy, presumably on the basis of an increase in noradrenergic activity. When it occurs, a reduction in dosage may help. We have been less impressed with the adjunctive use of bethanechol with MAOIs than with TCAs.

The most common side effect is dizziness, particularly of the orthostatic type. This appears to be somewhat more common with MAOIs than with TCAs. Dose reduction may help, but again we have often found this to be problematic, since too great a reduction in dose may lead to reemergence of depressive symptoms. Several approaches include 1) maintenance of adequate hydration—about eight glasses of fluid a day—and increased salt intake; 2) support stockings, bellybinders, or corsets; and 3) addition of a mineralocorti-

Table 3-7.   Common or troublesome side effects
of monoamine oxidase inhibitors

- Orthostatic hypotension
- Hypertensive crises (interactions with foodstuffs or medications)
- Hyperpyrexic reactions
- Anorgasmia or sexual impotence
- Sedation (particularly daytime and due to insomnia during night)
- Insomnia during night
- Stimulation during day
- Muscle cramps and myositis-like reactions
- Urinary hesitancy
- Constipation
- Dry mouth
- Weight gain
- Myoclonic twitches

coid (Florinef). Although this mineralocorticoid has been used in patients with orthostatic hypotension not induced by medication, we have rarely found it helpful in usual daily doses of 0.3 mg. We have been told by colleagues that Florinef can be effective at total daily doses of 0.6–0.8 mg. An intriguing report recently appeared pointing to the use of small amounts of cheese to help maintain blood pressure— a counterintuitive but imaginative solution. However, most clinicians are likely to be wary of the understandable risk of hypertensive crises with cheese, particularly when one does not really know the tyramine content of the foodstuff. Similarly, one would intuit that adding a stimulant (dextroamphetamine or methylphenidate) to an MAOI would result in marked surges of blood pressure. In fact, however, Feighner et al. (1985) reported that the addition of stimulants for patients receiving MAOIs or MAOI-TCA combinations normalized blood pressure in depressed patients with serious orthostatic hypotension, or brought out a clinical response in previously nonresponsive patients. There were no incidences of hypertensive crises; in fact, several of the patients developed orthostatic hypotension. Daily dosages used were 5–20 mg of *d*-amphetamine and 10–15 mg of methylphenidate. These authors recommend beginning at 2.5 mg/day of either drug. We have heard of several clinicians in the community who have used these approaches successfully, but we have also heard of at least one hypertensive crisis using stimulants in combination with MAOIs.

The greatest side-effect problems involve untoward interactions with certain foodstuffs or cold remedies, which may produce hypertensive crises with violent headaches and occasional cerebrovascular accidents, or hyperpyrexic states with myoclonus that can lead to coma. MAO in the intestinal tract degrades tyramine. When inhibited by MAOIs, the individual is at risk for absorbing large amounts of tyramine and probably other substances (e.g., phenylethylamine), which can act as false neurotransmitters or indirect agonists and elevate blood pressure. Fortunately, dietary restrictions can markedly reduce the risk. Various prohibited foods are included in lists in PDR. These lists have been reviewed by several investigators, and relative risks have been attributed to many of them (Table 3-8). As a general rule, we have begun to specifically advise patients to avoid eating in Chinese restaurants because of the ingredients used—soy sauce, sherry, etc.

Hyperpyrexic reactions are generally not due to interaction with foodstuffs. They generally represent increased central serotonin activity and may be particularly provoked by the addition of certain medications with potent serotonin reuptake–blocking properties, e.g., clomipramine or fluoxetine. In some cases of either hypertensive or hyperpyrexic reactions, the exact cause is not clear.

Of particular importance regarding medication interactions is warning patients *not* to take other medications along with the MAOIs without first checking with their physician. Demerol, epinephrine, local anesthetics (containing sympathomimetics), and decongestants can be particularly dangerous.

Frequently, we are asked which decongestant or antihistamine can be used with the MAOIs. Unfortunately, there is

Table 3-8. Foods to be avoided with monoamine oxidase inhibitors

---

- **Foods definitely to be avoided**
  Beer, red wine
  Aged cheeses (cottage and cream cheese are allowed)
  Dry sausage
  Fava or Italian green beans
  Brewer's yeast
  Smoked fish
  Liver (beef or chicken)

- **Foods that may cause problems in large amounts but are otherwise less problematic**
  Alcohol
  Ripe avocado
  Yogurt
  Bananas (ripe)
  ? Soy sauce

- **Foods that were thought to be problems but are probably not problematic in usual quantities**
  Chocolate
  Figs
  Meat tenderizers
  Caffeine-containing beverages
  Raisins

Source. Based on McCabe B, Tsuang MT: Dietary considerations in MAO inhibitor regimens. J Clin Psychiatry 43:178–181, 1982.

little in the way of prospective data. Diphenhydramine is used by many practitioners, with apparent success. One problem, however, with this approach is that some over-the-counter diphenhydramine elixirs contain pseudoephedrine, and at least one untoward interaction has been seen by our group. Another option is to use nasal sprays, but here, too, some patients may show increases in blood pressure.

Another issue has to do with surgery—emergency or otherwise—in patients treated with MAOIs. Although at first glance this seems a frightening prospect, there have been many patients who have successfully undergone surgery without consequence. Indeed, Dr. George Murray informed us that Massachusetts General Hospital has collected some 2,000 such cases. Obviously, anesthesiologists need to be apprised of a patient's medications so as to determine the safest approach. To this end, it is probably wise to have patients on MAOIs carry a Med-Alert card. Still, in many settings, surgeons and anesthesiologists will advise patients to go off MAOIs before undergoing surgery. Further study is needed to determine the most prudent approach to this knotty problem.

If a patient develops a surge in blood pressure with violent headaches, he or she should be instructed to go to a local emergency room. Phentolamine (Regitine), a central alpha blocker, can be administered intravenously to reverse the acute rise in blood pressure. Some psychopharmacologists have recommended that patients take oral chlorpromazine when headache occurs. We have tended not to do this if patients have not had a documented increase in blood pressure, because some patients will display marked head-aches secondary to a lowering of blood pressure. We have begun to provide our patients with nifedipine, a calcium channel blocker, in case they experience marked increases in blood pressure. Ten milligrams every hour until relief occurs (generally one or two doses) appears very helpful. This may prove problematic in elderly patients because acute lowering of blood pressure and myocardial infarction have been reported using this approach in older patients. We advise patients with headaches to have their blood pressure checked. Also, routine monitoring of blood pressure, particularly during the first 6 weeks of treatment with an MAOI, seems prudent (for both the drug's hypotensive and hypertensive effects).

Sedation and activation are also potential problems, the latter being more common. Activation takes two forms: stimulation during the day (particularly with tranylcypro-mine) and insomnia at night. Tranylcypromine's stimulatory effects have been related to its having a structure similar to that of amphetamines, although this pharmacologic link has not been clearly established. Overstimulation can be ameliorated somewhat by dose reduction, although the side effect is not easily eliminated. If a dose reduction does not result in a decrease in stimulation, patients may need to be switched to another medication.

Phenelzine overall is far less stimulating and more sedative than is tranylcypromine. As such it offers a major alternative for daytime overstimulation. However, phenelzine may produce both insomnia and secondary daytime sedation. Oddly, one often encounters insomnia in patients who are nevertheless showing a good clinical response, making it a particularly difficult side effect to manage. Changing the dosage regimen may be helpful. Patients who are not taking phenelzine in the evening may benefit from switching the drug to evening hours. Conversely, patients who are taking much of the drug in the evening may respond by taking it earlier in the day. These manipulations can be helpful, although in our experience they are highly variable in their efficacy. Some patients may ultimately require potent hypnotics to overcome persistent insomnia. We have been increasingly impressed with the addition of low doses of amitriptyline, trimipramine, or trazodone (50–100 mg at bedtime) to counteract MAOI-induced sleep disturbances. For trazodone, clinicians should adjust dose to avoid increased serotonergic activity and myoclonic jerks.

As the dose of an MAOI is increased to high levels in an attempt to achieve a therapeutic effect, patients occasionally become "intoxicated"—drunk, ataxic, confused, and sometimes euphoric. This is a sign of overdosage, and the dose should be reduced.

Some patients develop muscle pains or paresthesias which are probably the result of the MAOI interfering with pyridoxine (vitamin B_6) metabolism. Pyridoxine administered in doses of approximately 100 mg/day can be helpful.

A particularly bothersome side effect is anorgasmia, which

in some patients lessens over time. We have not been impressed with any pharmacologic attempts to counteract this side effect, although cyproheptadine (Periactin) has recently been said to be helpful. We have seen occasional patients helped with 4–8 mg taken an hour before sexual contact occurs.

If the clinician wishes to switch a patient from one MAOI to another, care must be taken to avoid drug-drug interactions. The clinician should taper the patient off one MAOI and allow for a 10- to 14-day drug-free period before beginning another MAOI. Some patients have experienced severe untoward reactions in switching from one MAOI to another, particularly from phenelzine to tranylcypromine, perhaps reflecting the latter's amphetamine-like properties.

When making a transition between TCAs and MAOIs, PDR recommends that patients be off all medications between trials for 10–14 days. Many clinicians, however, have reported that a briefer drug-free period of 1–5 days is sufficient when going from a TCA to an MAOI. When going from an MAOI to a TCA, the 10- to 14-day period is generally recommended. The difference in these strategies is probably due to the 10- to 14-day period needed to regenerate MAO. Thus, even after stopping MAOIs, patients should be warned to follow their dietary restrictions for an additional 14 days.

When transitioning between trazodone and MAOIs in either direction, a waiting period is not necessary. However, patients on MAOIs should wait 2 weeks before starting fluoxetine. When moving from fluoxetine to MAOIs, a 5-week period is recommended by the manufacturer because of the long half-life of the demethylated metabolite.

Augmenting Response

L-Tryptophan (2–6 g/day) added to MAOIs has been shown to improve or speed clinical response in a few studies. L-Tryptophan might also help as a mild hypnotic. However, we have not found that adding this amino acid is particularly helpful, and rare adverse effects suggestive of a serotonergic syndrome—such as tremor, myoclonic jerks, and confusion— have occurred in patients who are suddenly given 3–6 g of L-tryptophan on top of established MAOI therapy.

If a patient fails to respond to MAOIs, a trial of lithium may be added to induce a clinical response. Unlike the case of tricyclics, we have not found the addition of T_3 (Cytomel) helpful in augmenting clinical responsivity to MAOIs.

Selegiline (Eldepryl)

Selegiline was recently released by the FDA for use in Parkinson's disease under the trade name Eldepryl (see Figure 3-4). Much of the earlier clinical and scientific literature refers to selegiline by its earlier name, L-deprenyl.

At the doses used in Parkinson's disease, 5–10 mg a day, the drug is a selective inhibitor of MAO B, the form of the enzyme found in platelets and in some brain areas. MAO B does not metabolize norepinephrine; for this reason, it is believed that hypertensive crises should not occur with selegiline. Unfortunately, currently available studies of the use of L-deprenyl in depression suggest that doses of 15–60 mg/day are required to relieve depression. At these higher dosages, both MAO A and B are inhibited and hypertensive crises following ingestion of tyramine in foods seems likely. One such case, albeit mild, has been reported in a patient treated with 20 mg of selegiline a day. However, selegiline may ultimately prove to be safer than other available MAOIs in terms of the incidence and/or severity of hypertensive crises. It is simply too early to tell.

There are numerous published clinical studies of the drug in depression, the most recent ones being by Mann et al. (1989) at New York Hospital and by McGrath et al. (1989) at New York State Psychiatric Institute. These studies can be interpreted as confirming a clear therapeutic effect of selegiline in both atypical and endogenously depressed patients. The rate of clinical improvement is about 50%.

The drug is of substantial clinical interest because its pattern of side effects at doses up to 40 mg/day appears quite favorable when compared with the older MAOIs. Selegiline does not appear to cause clinically significant orthostatic hypotension or sexual dysfunction and may cause less insomnia than the older drugs. Several patients unable to tolerate the side effects of older MAOIs have tolerated selegiline quite well. It should be noted, however, that most published selegiline trials have lasted only 4–6 weeks, and some patients treated with the older MAOIs only develop clinically intolerable side effects after 2–3 months on the drug.

Among the several articles there are various preliminary findings about the kind of patients who do best (or least well) on L-deprenyl. Most of these are not confirmed by subsequent studies by the same group. One interesting suggestive pilot finding, not yet contradicted by further work, is that selegiline responders had dysphoric reactions to *d*-amphetamine before the study and low urinary MHPG levels. These suggestive findings are based on a sample of only eight patients (Liebowitz et al. 1985).

At this writing, selegiline (L-deprenyl) is a fascinating drug. It may turn out to be the best of the MAOIs—with fewer side effects and less risk of hypertensive crisis—but there is too little evidence to be sure of anything about the drug. Selegiline may be worth trying in treatment-resistant patients by psychiatrists already experienced in the management of patients on MAOIs. Patients with good antidepressant response to MAOIs but intolerable side effects may be the best candidates for selegiline.

Selegiline is not approved for use in depression, and patients should clearly understand the limited experience with the drug and give consent to its use. Because selegiline is metabolized to L-amphetamine and L-methamphetamine in the body and is a dopamine reuptake inhibitor, we strongly urge a 3-week interval between stopping an older MAOI and starting selegiline. All patients treated with selegiline should adhere to the full MAOI diet and medication avoidance program.

Two other comments are worth making. First, measuring platelet MAOIs in patients on selegiline is probably not useful since almost complete inhibition occurs after 1 week on 10 mg a day. Second, the drug is very expensive. A local drug store charges $2 per 5-mg pill.

TRAZODONE

Trazodone is a new breed of antidepressant introduced in Italy two decades ago and in the United States in 1981. It bears no structural resemblance to any of the other marketed antidepressants (Figure 3-5). However, it has a triazolo ring as does alprazolam (see Figure 6-1 in Chapter 6). It had been reported to be a central serotonin reuptake blocker as well as to have alpha norepinephrine receptor blocking effects. More recent studies indicate that it is primarily a blocker of $5\text{-}HT_1$ and $5\text{-}HT_2$ receptors. Its metabolite is a direct serotonin agonist. Its pharmacology is complex, and its specific mode of action has not been clearly described. Some clinicians have found the drug to be less potent than TCAs and MAOIs in endogenous depression. We have found it most effective in outpatients with mild to moderate depression and anxiety, particularly those with difficulty falling asleep.

The manufacturer recommends starting patients at 150 mg/day and then increasing up to 600 mg/day (Table 3-6). Our experience has been that the drug is quite sedating, and we begin patients at 50–100 mg/day and increase to 150 mg/day by days 3–5. Thereafter, we increase by 50–75 mg weekly to 300 mg/day. In our experience, patients respond at a modal dose of 150–300 mg/day. Indeed, some clinicians have proposed that trazodone has a therapeutic window; as with nortriptyline, too high plasma levels are associated with poor

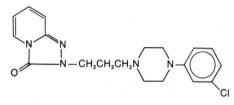

Trazodone

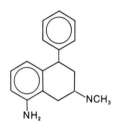

Nomifensine

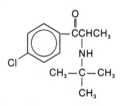

Bupropion

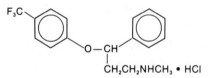

Fluoxetine

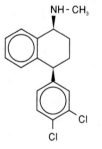

Sertraline

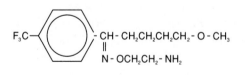

Fluvoxamine

Figure 3-5. Chemical structures of other antidepressants.

responses. Our experience would suggest this may be so, although the blood level studies done to date have not demonstrated any clear, rational relationships between blood levels and response.

We recently reviewed all studies that appeared after the drug was released in 1981 in which trazodone was compared with a known antidepressant or placebo. Of the nine studies, six included inpatients and eight included endogenously depressed patients. The drug was generally comparable to the tricyclic and significantly better than placebo. Those studies that reported poor results with trazodone used aggressive dosing, achieving doses of 300–450 mg/day in the first week. These data indicate that trazodone is an effective antidepressant and may be more effective at lower, rather than higher, dosages.

Trazodone is not anticholinergic. It can, however, produce dry mouth because of its alpha$_1$-receptor blockade. (Salivation is controlled by both acetylcholine and norepinephrine systems.) In addition to sedation, two side effects can be particularly troublesome. First, when taken on an empty stomach (particularly in high dosages), trazodone can produce acute dizziness and fainting. Patients should be warned to take the drug only after they have eaten. Some patients will also describe headaches or nausea rather than faintness if they take the drug on an empty stomach. Another reaction is priapism, with some 20 plus cases having been reported in the United States. This is rare but very problematic. Some patients may require surgical intervention. The acute treatment involves injection of an alpha agonist (e.g., epinephrine) into the penis. If not treated promptly, priapism may result in permanent impotence. Male patients should thus be warned to stop the drug immediately if they experience any symptoms suggestive of priapism (occasional erections are not problematic) and to seek emergency room treatment if the erection persists longer than 1 hour. Dr. Irwin Goldstein at Boston University Hospital has pioneered in treating this reaction and is a resource. Trazodone has a wide safety margin in cases of overdose.

Maintenance treatment with trazodone has been well studied in two trials. Patients have been reported to tolerate the drug well for prolonged periods. Generally, we have maintained patients at the dose to which they have responded.

TRIAZOLOBENZODIAZEPINES

Alprazolam

The triazolobenzodiazepine alprazolam is "approved" in patients with anxiety or anxiety associated with depression (see Figure 6-1 for chemical structure). However, the drug appears to have potent antipanic effects and only moderate antidepressant effects. Unlike diazepam or other typical benzodiazepines, alprazolam appears to affect noradrenergic systems (see Chapter 6) and to have reasonable effects comparable to imipramine and doxepin in mildly to moderately depressed outpatients at doses from 1.5 mg/day to as high as 6–10 mg/day. Generally, mildly to moderately depressed outpatients require 1.5–4.0 mg/day. We recommend starting at 1.0–1.5 mg/day, increasing the dosage by 0.5 mg every 3 days to 4.0 mg. The drug can be sedating, particularly in the patient previously not exposed to benzodiazepines. When stopping the drug, tapering is essential. Tapering is often done by a 0.5-mg reduction every 3 days. If the dosage is pushed too high and maintained for longer periods, discontinuation will take some time. This is a potential drawback to the drug (see Chapter 6).

Alprazolam's effects in seriously depressed endogenous patients are neither easily predicted nor consistent. It does appear to be an effective antidepressant in some patients with endogenous depression. For example, in one study of depressed inpatients with shortened rapid eye movement

(REM) latency, the drug was not as effective as amitriptyline but was effective in some patients. Because its effects in endogenous depression are so highly variable, its usefulness as a primary treatment in this group is limited. Mooney et al. (1985) reported that alprazolam enhances signal transduction by the receptor–N-protein–adenylate cyclase enzyme complex, and this effect may be related to drug response. But these tests are research tools and are not readily available.

Negative symptoms (anergia, withdrawal, etc.) are relatively common in schizophrenic patients. At times they are difficult to separate from depression or akinetic reactions to neuroleptics. There have been a few recent studies indicating that alprazolam may be useful in ameliorating negative symptoms in schizophrenic patients. There is one negative report, however. (For further discussion of alprazolam see Chapter 6.)

Adinazolam

Adinazolam (Deracyn) is another triazolobenzodiazepine with antidepressant properties. At this writing, it has not been released in the United States. Adinazolam has a half-life of 3 hours; its principal N-demethylated metabolite has a half-life of 4 hours. The drug appears to have greater activity than alprazolam in classic antidepressant animal paradigms. For example, it decreases forebrain serotonin activity and downregulates beta-receptors. Two reports of double-blind studies have been published, and the drug does appear to have antidepressant activity. In addition, adinazolam has been studied in inpatients and has comparable efficacy to that of amitriptyline and is significantly more effective than placebo. Both amitriptyline and adinazolam produced significantly greater reductions in the retardation factor of the Hamilton Rating Scale for Depression. However, because efficacy has not been clearly demonstrated in seriously suicidal patients and because of a possible risk of inducing disinhibition, the drug should not be used in such patients until further data are available to clarify if and when to use the drug in depressed patients.

The major side effect of adinazolam is sedation. It is used in doses of 30–120 mg/day. Even more than with alprazolam, adinazolam should be discontinued cautiously because of its short half-life. A sustained-release form is actively being studied to obviate this potential problem.

NOMIFENSINE

Nomifensine is a multicyclic compound (Figure 3-5) with both dopamine and norepinephrine reuptake blocking effects, conferring upon it both antidepressant and mild stimulant-like properties. It had been available in West Germany for many years, and European colleagues advocated it for the more anergic patient. We have seen several such patients who had failed to respond to TCAs but who responded very well to this compound. Its usual dosage range was 100–200 mg/day. The starting dose was 100 mg/day with 50 mg/day increases to 200–300 mg/day. Despite its short half-life (about 2 hours), studies indicated it could be given on a once-a-day basis, although twice-a-day administration (early morning and afternoon) was quite common.

Since the drug was often stimulating, patients were advised not to take the drug beyond the late afternoon. Additional side effects included agitation, sedation (in some patients), headaches, and insomnia. The drug appeared to have a reasonable safety margin in cases of overdosage, making it less problematic in suicidal patients. In addition, it did not appear to lower seizure thresholds. In a relatively small percentage of patients (as high as 3–10%), the drug produced an allergic reaction characterized by flulike symptoms and fever, not uncommonly seen with other quinoline compounds. Generally, this syndrome abated with discontinuation of the drug. It also produced mild elevations in blood pressure, particularly in patients on other sympathomimetic agents, as well as hemolytic anemia and elevations in liver enzymatic activity. The manufacturer recommended periodic blood counts and liver function tests in patients treated with the drug. However, because in Great Britain there had been a small number of deaths secondary to hemolytic anemias, the manufacturer discontinued the drug in early 1986. Although conceivably it could reappear on the U.S. market in the future, to date there has been no indication that this is likely to occur.

BUPROPION

Bupropion is a unicyclic (Figure 3-5) that was originally to be released in 1986, but was not released until mid-1989. This drug is neither a norepinephrine or a serotonin reuptake blocker. It does not inhibit monoamine oxidase. Its biochemical mode of action is unclear, although it has been hypothesized to act via dopamine reuptake blockade. This remains moot since its dopamine potentiating effects in animals appear to occur at very high dosages and blood levels, well beyond those expected in humans. Moreover, when dopamine effects were demonstrated in humans in one study, they appeared to be related to possible psychotic reactions to the drug rather than to its antidepressant responses. The drug appears effective in patients with depression. One pilot study of bupropion in panic disorder was quite negative (Sheehan et al. 1983); more recent informal clinical experience suggests that some treatment-resistant panic patients respond well.

Bupropion has a relatively wide usual dosage range of 200–450 mg/day (see Table 3-6). The modal optimum dosage range in our experience has been 300–400 mg/day. Bupropion is available in 15-mg and 100-mg tablets; a 50-mg tablet is in preparation.

Bupropion has a favorable side-effect profile since it is not anticholinergic. Its side effects have appeared to us to be nonspecific in the patients we have treated over the past few years, although nausea occurs in occasional patients. It does not induce orthostatic hypotension or stimulate appetite. Some investigators have argued that the drug could be particularly useful in patients who gain weight while taking TCAs. There are reports that patients with sexual dysfunction on other antidepressants do better on bupropion. Seizures had been reported at the rate of 3 per 1,000 at doses less than 450 mg/day. The occurrence of seizures in a study on bulimic patients led to a delay in the expected release of the drug in 1986 pending a large-scale study to determine more precisely the risk of seizures in depressed patients. This study has been completed and the data have been analyzed. The prevalence of seizures was no higher than previously found. Because of the potential risk of seizures in certain patient populations, the manufacturer recommends the drug not be given to patients with any history of seizures, major head injury, bulimia, or anorexia nervosa. The manufacturer also cautions that single doses of the drug should never exceed 150 mg. There are suggestions that the drug is less likely to produce mania, and it appears safe in overdoses.

SEROTONIN REUPTAKE BLOCKERS

Fluoxetine

Fluoxetine (Prozac) is one of a new group of antidepressant drugs that selectively inhibit the reuptake of serotonin. Its chemical structure is depicted in Figure 3-5. The drug was released early in 1988.

Fluoxetine exerts little effect on norepinephrine or dopamine reuptake in rat brain synaptosomes. In contrast, it is a potent serotonin reuptake blocker; its serotonin reuptake blocking effects are approximately 100 times those of norepinephrine or dopamine reuptake. The drug is 15–60 times more potent as a serotonin reuptake blocker than is amitriptyline or doxepin. In contrast to fluoxetine's selective serotonin reuptake effects, amitriptyline and doxepin in similar models are at best equipotent in their norepinephrine and serotonin activity. In other models, they exert virtually no effect on serotonin but rather affect norepinephrine reuptake blockade selectively. Fluoxetine potently antagonizes brain serotonin—but not cardiac norepinephrine—depletion in mice treated with p-chloramphetamine and 6-OH-dopamine, respectively. Interestingly, in this same model, amitriptyline, doxepin, and trazodone did not reverse serotonin depletion, although they did exert serotonin reuptake blocking effects in the rat brain synaptosome model described above. Fluoxetine exerts very little effect on blocking muscarinic anticholinergic, histamine (H_1), serotonin ($5\text{-}HT_1$ and $5\text{-}HT_2$), and alpha$_1$ and alpha$_2$ norepinephrine receptors.

Fluoxetine's half-life is approximately 1–3 days; that of its demethylated metabolite, 7–9 days. It does not alter the pharmacokinetic properties of anticonvulsants, chlorthiazide, or possibly diazepam, nor does it increase blood concentrations of ethanol. Psychometric studies indicate that it does not enhance ethanol's effects on neurometric or psychomotor performance. There are several case reports that fluoxetine increases TCA blood levels substantially when combined with TCAs. Recent studies indicate that fluoxetine may significantly increase the plasma levels of diazepam and alprazolam (Lemberger et al. 1988; The Upjohn Company 1990). (For further discussion see Chapter 9.)

A number of double-blind studies have demonstrated fluoxetine to be of equal efficacy to doxepin, amitriptyline, and desipramine, and to be significantly more effective than placebo, in the treatment of outpatients with major depression. In our previous edition, we discussed the expected dosage schedule that had been used in the double-blind studies. That protocol called for the drug to be initiated at 20 mg/day with increases to 40 mg/day for days 2–4 and 60 mg/day on days 5–7. The maximum recommended daily dosage of 80 mg/day could be attained by day eight. A review of the double-blind efficacy data revealed that fluoxetine produced maximal benefits at 20–40 mg/day with lesser benefit noted at 60 and 80 mg/day. In fact, 80 mg appeared to produce less efficacy and greater side effects. Because 20 mg was often effective and the drug has a long half-life, the manufacturer altered the recommended dosing to 20 mg/day for 3 weeks with subsequent increases to 40–80 mg/day. In many patients, 10 mg/day is effective as well. The drug is currently available only in 20-mg capsules. In patients requiring less than 20 mg/day (e.g., those with pronounced side effects), 20 mg can be given on an every-other-day schedule or the contents of the capsule can be dissolved in water or juice and half taken daily. The fluoxetine-containing juice should be refrigerated.

In an interesting study, Reimherr and colleagues (1984) reported that patients with chronic and refractory depressions responded more favorably to fluoxetine than to imipramine. The two drugs were equal in more typical, episodic depressive patients. Thus, fluoxetine appears to be a major alternative to previously available compounds.

Fluoxetine's side-effect profile is generally more favorable than that of the TCAs. It produces much less in the way of orthostatic hypotension, constipation, and dry mouth, appearing quite similar to placebo in the incidence of these side reactions. Its major side effects are nausea, tremor, drowsiness, sweating, headache, and nervousness. A common question is whether one can prescribe the drug in anxious depressive patients. An analysis of double-blind studies indicates the drug can be effective for such patients, although concomitant treatment with an anxiolytic or hypnotic may be required. In 110 patients studied at McLean Hospital before the drug's release, higher baseline levels of anxiety and insomnia were associated with slightly more improvement on treatment with fluoxetine.

Unlike most tricyclics, fluoxetine appears to facilitate weight loss acutely. We have, however, seen several patients who initially lost weight on the drug but who regained that weight (and then some) while on maintenance treatment. Most patients have been able to maintain their weight loss. We have seen a few women with a history of bruising who appeared to bruise even more easily after receiving this drug. The extent of the problem has to date not been marked.

Fluoxetine appears relatively safe in overdosages. One fatality was reported in the early clinical trials in a patient who had also taken a number of other potentially lethal substances. There have been a few overdoses in the clinical trials on fluoxetine alone, but none of these reportedly resulted in fatality. There has been one recent fatality ascribed to an overdose of fluoxetine alone. Thus, the drug appears to offer an advantage over TCAs and MAOIs, although broader clinical use will ultimately be needed to fully map out its side-effect profile and limits of safety. Teicher et al. (1990) reported the emergence of intense preoccupation with suicide in six patients early in fluoxetine treatment. This may also occur with other antidepressants. Despite recent intense media attention paid to this problem, clinicians should mainly be aware that it can occur. This suicidality abates fairly rapidly once the drug is stopped. Some patients who experience this phenomenon on a TCA may not experience it with fluoxetine.

One potential problem that has emerged is an untoward interaction of fluoxetine with MAOIs, particularly the development of a serotonergic syndrome. Two deaths were reported in patients whose fluoxetine was stopped but who were promptly begun on MAOIs. It is unclear whether other factors were also involved in these two cases; however, the manufacturer has recommended waiting 5 weeks when going from fluoxetine to an MAOI. This period is five times the half-life of the active metabolite of fluoxetine. It is conceivable that a shorter period (e.g., 3 weeks) may suffice, but no data are available. When going from an MAOI to fluoxetine, 2 weeks off MAOIs are recommended. In addition, myoclonic jerks have been reported in patients treated with fluoxetine combined with L-tryptophan, and this combination is also contraindicated.

Fluoxetine is being actively studied for the treatment of a number of conditions, particularly bulimia, obsessive-compulsive disorder, and obesity. The drug appears effective in bulimic patients. Its antiobsessive properties are being investigated, but data to date are limited. The drug appears to promote considerable weight loss (about 8–10 lbs) in an 8-week period in obese patients; however, follow-up studies suggest subjects may regain their weight over 6 months in the absence of other treatments. Alcohol consumption has reportedly been reduced in lower animals and humans by the administration of L-tryptophan or serotonin reuptake blockers including fluoxetine. In problem drinkers, serotonin reuptake blockers result in less frequent consumption but do not ablate it. There have been two reports of fluoxetine being helpful in patients with borderline personality disorder. At any rate, fluoxetine (and other serotonin reuptake blockers) appear to have great potential for treating a variety of conditions. It is likely that dosing schedules will be different for these other conditions. For example, obese and bulimic patients appear to require approximately 60 mg/day. These indications may require higher-strength formulations—e.g., a 60-mg capsule.

Fluvoxamine

Fluvoxamine is another specific serotonin reuptake blocker. It is widely available in Europe and in this country has been studied in depression and obsessive-compulsive disorder. Early double-blind studies in the United States and Canada did not show fluvoxamine or frequently the comparison TCAs to be particularly effective in depression. These studies tended to be of relatively short duration (about 4 weeks) in outpatients. When some of these studies were extended to 5–6 weeks, fluvoxamine appeared to have clearer antidepressant properties. Recently completed studies—many not yet in print at the time of our writing—are apparently finding the drug to be effective, although the European experience suggests the drug may be a weaker antidepressant than some other serotonin reuptake blockers. In early North American studies, the incidence of nausea with other serotonin reuptake blockers was much higher (up to 50%) than that reported for fluoxetine. The drug has been studied in obsessive-compulsive disorder, and these studies indicate the drug is effective in this condition (see Chapter 6).

Other Serotonergic Antidepressants

There are a number of serotonergic agents under study in the United States and abroad. These agents can be roughly divided into serotonin reuptake blockers and serotonin agonists. Of the former class, sertraline is the compound other than fluvoxamine that is closest to being released in the United States. This drug appears to have antidepressant efficacy and to have a somewhat better side-effect profile than other drugs of its class. Citalopram is a European drug whose U.S. career was halted because of possible toxicity in primates. Of the agonists, gepirone, which acts on 5-HT_{1A} receptors, is under active investigation, and preliminary studies have reportedly been favorable. There are a number of other agonists currently being tested in the United States and abroad. For example, buspirone, a serotonin agonist marketed for anxiety, is being studied at higher dosages as an antidepressant.

Bibliography

Amsterdam JD, Berwish NJ: High dose tranylcypromine therapy for refractory depression. Pharmacopsychiatry 22:21–25, 1989

Aranow RB, Hudson JL, Pope HG, et al: Elevated antidepressant plasma levels after addition of fluoxetine. Am J Psychiatry 146:911–913, 1989

Asberg M, Cronholm B, Sjoqvist F, et al: Relationship between plasma level and therapeutic effect of nortriptyline. Br Med J 3:331–334, 1971

Baron BM, Ogden AM, Seigel BW, et al: Rapid down-regulation of beta-adrenoreceptors by co-administration of desipramine and fluoxetine. Eur J Pharmacol 154:125–134, 1988

Beaumont G: The toxicity of antidepressants. Br J Psychiatry 154:454–458, 1989

Bell IR, Cole JO: Fluoxetine induces elevation of desipramine levels and exacerbation of geriatric nonpsychotic depression (letter). J Clin Psychopharmacol 8:447–448, 1988

Bielski RJ, Friedel RO: Prediction of tricyclic antidepressant response: a critical review. Arch Gen Psychiatry 33:1479–1489, 1976

Cohen B, Harris P, Altesman R: Amoxapine: neuroleptic as well as an antidepressant? Am J Psychiatry 139:1165–1167, 1982

Cohn JP, Wilcox C: A comparison of fluoxetine, imipramine, and placebo in patients with major depressive disorder. J Clin Psychiatry 46(3, sec 2):26–31, 1985

Cole JO, Bodkin JA: Antidepressant drug side effects. J Clin Psychiatry 51 (suppl 1):21–26, 1990

Cole JO, Schatzberg AF: Antidepressant drug therapy, in Psychiatry Update: The American Psychiatric Association Annual Review, Vol 2. Edited by Grinspoon L. Washington, DC, American Psychiatric Press, 1983, pp 472–491, 542–544

Cooper GL: The safety of fluoxetine—an update. Br J Psychiatry 153 (suppl 3):77–86, 1988

Dessain EC, Schatzberg AF, Woods BT, et al: Maprotiline treatment in depression: a perspective on seizures. Arch Gen Psychiatry 43:86–90, 1986

Feighner JP, Aden GC, Fabre LF, et al: Comparison of alprazolam, imipramine and placebo in the treatment of depression. JAMA 249:3056–3064, 1983

Feighner JP, Herbstein J, Damlouji N: Combined MAOI, TCA, and direct stimulant therapy of treatment-resistant depression. J Clin Psychiatry 46:206–209, 1985

For Refractory Depression: Rx High-Dose MAOI? Biological Therapies in Psychiatry Newsletter 12:25, 28, 1989

Gardner E: Long-term preventive care in depression: the use of bupropion in patients intolerant of other antidepressants. J Clin Psychiatry 44:163–169, 1983

Glassman AH, Perel JM, Shostak M, et al: Clinical implications of imipramine plasma levels for depressive illness. Arch Gen Psychiatry 34:197–204, 1977

Joyce PR, Paykel ES: Predictors of drug response in depression. Arch Gen Psychiatry 46:89–99, 1989

Kline NS: Clinical experience with iproniazid (Marsilid). Journal of Clinical and Experimental Psychopathology 19:72–78, 1958

Kocsis JH, Cronghan JL, Katz MM, et al: Response to treatment with antidepressants of patients with severe or moderate nonpsychotic depression and of patients with psychotic depression. Am J Psychiatry 117:621–624, 1990

Kuhn R: Uber die behandlung depressiver zustande mit einem iminodibenzylderivat (G22355). Schweiz Med Wochenschr 87:1135–1140, 1957

Lemberger L, Bergstrom RF, Wolen RL, et al: Fluoxetine: Clinical pharmacology and physiology disposition. J Clin Psychiatry 46(3, sec 2):14–19, 1985

Lemberger L, Rowe H, Bosomworth J, et al: The effect of fluoxetine on the pharmacokinetics and psychomotor responses of diazepam. Clin Pharmacol Ther 43:412–419, 1988

Liebowitz M, Karoun F, Quitkin F: Biochemical effects of 1-deprenyl in atypical depressives. Biol Psychiatry 20:558–565, 1985

Liebowitz MR, Quitkin FM, Stewart JW: Antidepressant specificity in atypical depression. Arch Gen Psychiatry 45:129–137, 1988

Mangla JC, Pereira M: Tricyclic antidepressants in the treatment of peptic ulcer disease. Arch Intern Med 142:273–275, 1982

Mann JJ, Aarons SF, Wilner PJ, et al: A controlled study of the antidepressant efficacy and side effects of (−)-deprenyl: a selective monoamine oxidase inhibitor. Arch Gen Psychiatry 46:45–50, 1989

McCabe B, Tsuang MT: Dietary consideration in MAO inhibitor regimens. J Clin Psychiatry 43:178–181, 1982

McGrath PJ, Quitkin FM, Harrison W, et al: Treatment of melancholia with tranylcypromine. Am J Psychiatry 141:288–289, 1984

McGrath PJ, Stewart JW, Harrison W, et al: A placebo-controlled trial of 1-deprenyl in atypical depression. Psychopharmacol Bull 25:63–67, 1989

Mirin SM, Schatzberg AF, Creasey DE: Hypomania and mania after tricyclic withdrawal. Am J Psychiatry 138:87–89, 1981

Monoamine oxidase inhibitors and anesthesia: an update. International Drug Therapy Newsletter 24:13–14, 1989

Mooney JJ, Schatzberg AF, Cole JO, et al: Enhanced signal transduction by adenylate cyclase in platelet membranes of patients showing antidepressant responses to alprazolam: preliminary data. J Psychiatr Res 19:65–75, 1985

Naranjo CA, Sellers EM: Research Advances in New Psychopharmacological Treatments for Alcoholism. New York, Excerpta Medica, 1985

Nelson JC, Shottenfeld RS, Conrad CD: Hypomania after desipramine withdrawal. Am J Psychiatry 140:624–625, 1983

Nierenberg AA, Keck PE: Management of monoamine oxidase inhibition associated insomnia with trazodone. J Clin Psychopharmacol 9:42–45, 1989

Nordern MJ: Fluoxetine in borderline personality disorder. Prog Neuro-Psychopharmacol Biol Psychiatry 13:885–893, 1989

Pearlstein T, Frances AJ, Kocsis JH, et al: A controlled study of the antidepressant efficacy and side effects of (−)-deprenyl, a selective monoamine oxidase inhibitor. Arch Gen Psychiatry 46:45–50, 1989

Pope HG, Hudson JI, Jonas JM, et al: Bulimia treated with imipramine: a placebo-controlled, double-blind study. Am J Psychiatry 140:554–558, 1983

Prien RF, Kupfer DJ, Mansky PA, et al: Drug therapy in the prevention of recurrences in unipolar and bipolar affective disorders. Arch Gen Psychiatry 41:1096–1104, 1984

Quitkin F, Rabkin A, Klein DF: Monoamine oxidase inhibitors. Arch Gen Psychiatry 36:749–760, 1979

Quitkin FM, Rabkin JG, Ross D, et al: Duration of antidepressant drug treatment: what is an adequate trial? Arch Gen Psychiatry 41:238–245, 1984

Rappoport JL, Mikkelsen EJ, Zavadil A, et al: Childhood enuresis, II: psychopathology, tricyclic concentration in plasma and antienuretic effect. Arch Gen Psychiatry 37:1146–1152, 1980

Ravaris CL, Nies A, Robinson DS, et al: A multiple-dose controlled study of phenelzine in depression-anxiety states. Arch Gen Psychiatry 33:347–350, 1976

Reinherr FW, Wood DR, Byerley B, et al: Characteristics of responders to fluoxetine. Psychopharmacol Bull 20:70–72, 1984

Richelson E: The use of tricyclic antidepressants in chronic gastrointestinal pain. J Clin Psychiatry 43:50–55, 1982

Richelson E: Synaptic pharmacology of antidepressants: an update. McLean Hospital Journal 13:67–88, 1988

Richelson E, Nelson A: Antagonism by antidepressants of neurotransmitter receptors of normal human brain in vitro. J Pharmacol Exp Ther 230:94–102, 1984

Rickels K, Chung HR, Csanolsi IB, et al: Alprazolam, diazepam, imipramine, and placebo in outpatients with major depression. Arch Gen Psychiatry 44:862–866, 1987

Robinson DS, Nies A, Ravaris CL, et al: Clinical pharmacology of phenelzine. Arch Gen Psychiatry 35:629–635, 1978

Robinson DS, Kayser A, Corcella J, et al: Hyperphagia, hypersomnia, panic attacks, hysterical traits, and somatic anxiety predict phenelzine response in depressed outpatients. Presented at the annual meeting of the American College of Neuropsychopharmacology, San Juan, Puerto Rico, December 1983

Roose SP, Glassman AH: Cardiovascular effects of tricyclic antidepressants in depressed patients. J Clin Psychiatry Monograph Series 7(No 2):1–18, 1989

Sargant W: The treatment of anxiety states and atypical depressions by the monoamine oxidase inhibitor drugs. J Neuropsychiatry 3 (suppl 1):96–103, 1962

Schatzberg AF: Triazolobenzodiazepines in the treatment of depressive disorders, in Proceedings of the British Association for Psychopharmacology—Thirty Years On. Edited by Leonard B. London, CNS Publishers, 1990

Schatzberg AF, Cole JO: Benzodiazepines in depressive disorders. Arch Gen Psychiatry 35:1359–1365, 1978

Schatzberg AF, Cole JO, Blumer DP: Speech blockage: a tricyclic side effect. Am J Psychiatry 135:600–601, 1978

Schatzberg AF, Rosenbaum AH, Orsulak PJ, et al: Toward a biochemical classification of depressive disorders, III: pretreatment urinary MHPG levels as predictors of response to maprotiline. Psychopharmacology 75:34–38, 1981

Schatzberg AF, Cole JO, Cohen BM, et al: Survey of depressed patients who have failed to respond to treatment, in Affective Disorders. Edited by Davis JM, Maas J. Washington, DC, American Psychiatric Press, 1983

Sheehan DV, Davidson J, Manshreck TC, et al: Lack of efficacy of a new antidepressant (bupropion) in the treatment of panic disorder with phobias. J Clin Psychopharmacol 3:23–31, 1983

Shopsin B: Bupropion's prophylactic efficacy in bipolar affective illness. J Clin Psychiatry 44:163–169, 1983

Spiegel K, Kalb R, Pasternak GW: Analgesic activity of tricyclic antidepressants. Ann Neurol 13:462–465, 1983

Spiker DG, Hanin I, Cofsky J, et al: Pharmacological treatment of delusional depressives. Psychopharmacol Bull 17:201–202, 1981

Stark P, Fuller RW, Wong DT: The pharmacologic profile of fluoxetine. J Clin Psychiatry 46(3, sec 2):7–13, 1985

Stewart JW, Harrison W, Quitkin FM, et al: Phenelzine-induced pyridoxine deficiency. J Clin Psychopharmacol 4:225–226, 1984

Sunderland T, Cohen RM, Thompson KE, et al: L-Deprenyl treatment of older depressives (NR-159), in New Research Program and Abstracts. Washington, DC, American Psychiatric Association, 1989

Switching MAOI's [Newsnote]. Biological Therapies in Psychiatry 7(9):33–36, 1984

Teicher MH, Cohen BM, Baldessarini RJ, et al: Severe daytime somnolence in patients treated with an MAOI. Am J Psychiatry 145:1552–1556, 1988

Teicher MH, Glod C, Cole JO: Emergence of intense suicidal preoccupation during fluoxetine treatment. Am J Psychiatry 147:207–210, 1990

Treatment of xerostomia. Med Lett Drugs Ther 30:74–76, 1988

Tyrer P: Towards rational therapy with monoamine oxidase inhibitors. Br J Psychiatry 128:354–360, 1976

The Upjohn Company: Technical report synopsis: a pharmacokinetic/pharmacodynamic evaluation of the combined administration of alprazolam and fluoxetine. Kalamazoo, MI, The Upjohn Company, 1990

Walsh BT, Stewart JW, Wright L, et al: Treatment of bulimia with monoamine oxidase inhibitors. Am J Psychiatry 139:1629–1630, 1982

Wander TJ, Nelson A, Okazaki H: Antagonism by antidepressants of serotonin S1 and S2 receptors of normal human brain in vitro. Eur J Pharmacol 132:115–121, 1986

Warrington SJ, Padgham C, Lader M: The cardiovascular effects of antidepressants (Psychological Medicine, Monograph Supplement 16). Cambridge, Cambridge University Press, 1989

Weilburg JB, Rosenbaum JF, Biederman J, et al: Fluoxetine added to non-MAOI antidepressants converts nonresponders to responders: a preliminary report. J Clin Psychiatry 50:447–449, 1989

Wernicke JF: The side effect profile and safety of fluoxetine. J Clin Psychiatry 46(3, sec 2):59–67, 1985

Antipsychotic Drugs

4

In 1952, chlorpromazine was developed as an antiautonomic drug to protect the body against its own excessive compensatory reactions during major surgery. It spread into psychiatry from the field of anesthesia, after an initial clinical report by Delay et al. (1952) demonstrated the drug's good features and its efficacy in acute psychosis. Endless subsequent double-blind studies have served chiefly to confirm the effects already obvious to the original French clinicians.

We now know substantially more about the side effects and limitations of the currently available antipsychotic drugs and more about their mechanisms of action. We are beginning to understand dose-response relationships and finally have generally available a somewhat more effective atypical neuroleptic, clozapine, for use in treatment-resistant patients.

THE DRUGS

There are, at the time of writing, 15 antipsychotic drugs available for prescription use in the United States: 8 pheno-

thiazines, 2 thioxanthenes, 2 dibenzazepines, 2 butyrophenones, and an indole (Table 4-1, Figure 4-1). One of these,
pimozide, is approved for use only in Gilles de la Tourette's
syndrome, but it is almost certainly an effective antipsychotic.
All but 3 of the 16 are variants on the three-ring phenothiazine
structure, and all are reasonably potent postsynaptic dopamine receptor blockers (dopamine antagonists). Although it
is conceivable that these drugs might act in psychosis by
some other mechanism, it seems unlikely. The only other
available type of drug with some documented efficacy in
schizophrenia, reserpine, presumably works to reduce dopaminergic brain activity by depleting cells of dopamine
instead of blocking receptors. Only one clinically proven
antipsychotic dibenzazepine—clozapine—*may* work by a different mechanism. Other drugs such as lithium carbonate
and carbamazepine (see Chapter 5) and propranolol, diazepam, and alprazolam (see Chapter 6) have been shown to
ameliorate schizophrenic symptoms under some circumstances in some patients, but none of these have clear, proven
efficacy at all comparable to the standard antipsychotics.

All the effective antipsychotic drugs, except clozapine, act
on the nigrostriatal system in the predicted manner, producing
pseudoparkinsonism. The clinically useful dosages of the
various antipsychotic drugs correlate best with their ability
to block dopamine-2 receptors. Neither clinical usefulness
nor side effects relate at all sensibly to the varying abilities
of clinically prescribable drugs to affect dopamine-1 versus
dopamine-2 receptors. There are no pure dopamine-1 or -2
drugs available for clinical use. It is presumed, but by no
means proven, that the antipsychotics ameliorate schizophrenia by acting on mesolimbic or mesocortical dopamine
systems. The drugs also have endocrine effects through
dopamine receptors in the hypothalamic-pituitary axis. Of
these, only the endocrine and nigrostriatal effects are at all
helpful in understanding the clinical use of the drugs and
then only in explaining and treating common side effects. As

far as the major clinical action of the standard antipsychotic drugs are concerned, they could equally well be conceived to be working on the pineal gland or the psyche. Unfortunately, we do not as yet have an effective, safe antipsychotic without parkinsonian and related side effects.

Even though clozapine, with its risk of agranulocytosis, has been known to be unique in its action on psychosis for over 10 years and to be relatively free of parkinsonian side effects, no comparable drug has been discovered to replace it despite the efforts of many major pharmaceutical firms. Clozapine has been available in some foreign countries and is now available in the United States. Other investigational antipsychotics are under clinical trial in the United States; however, a wide variety of other antipsychotics are generally available in European countries. This chapter will consider standard antipsychotics, clozapine, and pimozide and briefly discuss foreign antipsychotics.

EFFICACY

All the available standard antipsychotic drugs have been clearly shown to be more effective than placebo in schizophrenia, both acute and chronic. Most major studies were done many years ago using some variant of the DSM-II criteria and involved an unknown but possibly large proportion of acute patients who might be judged schizophreniform or atypical bipolar or schizoaffective by current DSM-III-R standards. It is, therefore, clinically sensible to assume that all the drugs are effective in all these DSM-III-R conditions and to include mania as a proven indication as well. Since the studies of chronic patients surely contained mainly DSM-III-R schizophrenic patients, there is little doubt that "real" schizophrenia responds to antipsychotic drugs as well.

In many respects, the nature and timing of clinical response to antipsychotics is unsatisfactory. In large-scale 6-week placebo-controlled trials in hospitalized patients, 75% of

Table 4-1. Antipsychotic drugs

Generic name	Brand name	Dosage forms
chlorpromazine	Thorazine*	Tablet: 10, 25, 50, 100, 200 mg Spansule: 30, 75, 150, 200, 300 mg Suppository: 25, 100 mg Syrup: 10 mg/5 ml (4-oz bottle) Concentrate: 30 mg/ml (4-oz bottle), 100 mg/ml (8-oz bottle) Ampule: 25 mg/ml (1 ml, 2 ml) Multidose vial: 25 mg/ml (10 ml)
chlorprothixene	Taractan	Tablet: 10, 25, 50, 100 mg Concentrate: 100 mg/5 ml (16-oz bottle) Ampule: 25 mg/2 ml
clozapine	Clozaril†	Tablet: 25, 100 mg
droperidol	Inapsine*	Ampule: 2.5 mg/ml (1, 2, 5 ml) Vial: 2.5 mg/ml 10 ml (1)
fluphenazine HCl	Permitil	Tablet: 2.5, 5, 10 mg Concentrate: 5 mg/ml (4-oz bottle)
	Prolixin*	Tablet: 1, 2.5, 5, 10 mg Concentrate: 5 mg/ml (4-oz bottle) Elixir: 2.5 mg/5 ml (16-oz bottle) Parenteral: 2.5 mg/ml (10-ml vial)
fluphenazine decanoate	Prolixin decanoate*	Syringe: 2.5 mg/ml (1 ml) Vial: 5 ml

fluphenazine enanthate	Prolixin enanthate	Syringe: 25 mg/ml Vial: 5 ml
haloperidol	Haldol*	Tablet: 0.5, 1, 2, 5, 10, 20 mg Concentrate: 2 mg/ml (15-ml, 120-ml, and 480-ml bottle) Parenteral: 5 mg/ml Ampule: 1 ml Syringe (disposable): 1 ml Vial: 10 ml
haloperidol decanoate	Haldol*	Ampule: 50 mg/ml (1 ml), 100 mg/ml‡
loxapine	Loxitane	Capsule: 5, 10, 25, 50 mg Concentrate: 25 mg/ml (120-ml bottle) Parenteral: 50 mg/ml Vial: 1 ml/10 ml
mesoridazine	Serentil	Tablet: 10, 25, 50, 100 mg Concentrate: 25 mg/ml (4-oz bottle) Ampule: 25 mg/ml (1 ml)
molindone	Moban	Tablet: 5, 10, 25, 50, 100 mg Concentrate: 20 mg/ml (120-ml bottle)
perphenazine	Trilafon*	Tablet: 2, 4, 8, 16 mg Repetab: 8 mg Concentrate: 16 mg/5 ml (4-oz bottle) Ampule: 5 mg/ml (1 ml)
pimozide	Orap	Tablet: 2 mg

Table 4-1. Antipsychotic drugs (*continued*)

Generic name	Brand name	Dosage forms
prochlorperazine	Compazine*	Tablet: 5, 10, 25 mg Spansule: 10, 15, 30 mg Suppository: 2.5, 5, 25 mg Syrup: 5 mg/5 ml (4-oz bottle) Parenteral: 5 mg/ml Ampule: 2 ml Syringe (disposable): 1 ml, 2 ml Vial: 10 ml (multidose)
thioridazine	Mellaril*	Tablet: 10, 15, 25, 50, 100, 150, 200 mg Concentrate: 30 mg/ml (4-oz bottle), 100 mg/ml (16-oz bottle) Suspension: 25 mg/5 ml, 100 mg/5 ml (16-oz bottle)
thiothixene	Navane*	Capsule: 1, 2, 5, 10, 20 mg Concentrate: 5 mg/ml (1-oz bottle, 4-oz bottle) Parenteral: 2 mg/ml, 5 mg/ml Vial: 2 mg
trifluoperazine	Stelazine*	Tablet: 1, 2, 5, 10 mg Concentrate: 10 mg/ml (2-oz bottle) Parenteral: 2 mg/ml Vial: 10 ml

* Available in generic form.
† Available only through the CPMS (Clozaril Patient Management System).
‡ The 100 mg/ml form of Haldol is not available generically.

A. PHENOTHIAZINES

1. Aliphatic

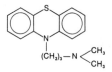

Promazine

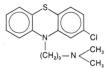

Chlorpromazine

Triflupromazine

2. Piperidine

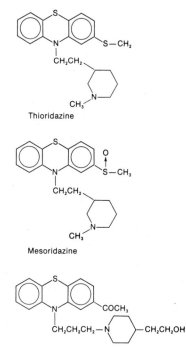

Thioridazine

Mesoridazine

Piperacetazine

Figure 4-1. Chemical structures of antipsychotic drugs.

drug-treated patients showed at least moderate improvement, whereas only 25% of placebo-treated patients did as well, and some got worse. However, many patients never achieve complete remission, and few are able to function at a fully effective level upon return to the community.

Antipsychotic drugs are also relatively unsatisfactory as maintenance therapy. In one major study, one-half of the antipsychotic-treated schizophrenic patients relapsed over the 2-year study period. About 85% of the placebo-treated patients relapsed over the same period. It thus appears that

3. Piperazine

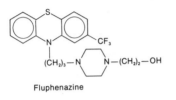

Fluphenazine

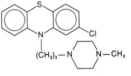

Prochlorperazine

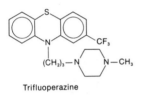

Trifluoperazine

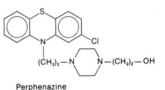

Perphenazine

Figure 4-1. Chemical structures of antipsychotic drugs (*continued*).

antipsychotics are more effective than placebo, but many patients relapse despite adequate drug therapy.

Further, the drugs tend to act in a slow, approximate manner. A few patients show rapid, excellent response, but most get better more slowly and some do not respond at all or do so only very slowly. Sometimes the response is so slow and variable as to encourage the prescribing of very high drug dosages early in treatment in an understandable but probably misguided effort to speed clinical response.

In recent studies as well as in studies done 20 years ago, improvement increases relatively rapidly between the 1st and 6th week on the drug. Thereafter, modest further improvement occurs between the 6th and 13th week, with a little

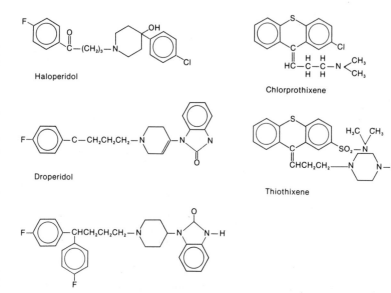

B. BUTYROPHENONE-LIKE

Haloperidol

Droperidol

Pimozide

C. THIOXANTHENES

Chlorprothixene

Thiothixene

Figure 4-1. Chemical structures of antipsychotic drugs (*continued*).

additional improvement by the 26th week. These changes are, of course, average improvement figures—individual patients may improve more or less, earlier or later. Similarly, once a patient is better, it is difficult to find the minimal effective maintenance dose in any reliable way. One might imagine that the physician could gradually reduce the dose from that on which the patient had recovered (e.g., 20 mg of haloperidol a day) by 2 mg a week until psychotic symptoms began to reemerge (e.g., at 4 mg a day) and then raise the dose a little until the patient is restabilized; the final dose (e.g., 6 mg a day) would then be the minimal effective maintenance dose. Unfortunately, when stable patients are shifted from an antipsychotic drug to placebo abruptly, they

D. INDOLE

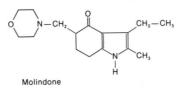

Molindone

E. DIBENZAZEPINE

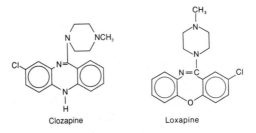

Clozapine　　　　　　　　Loxapine

Figure 4-1. Chemical structures of antipsychotic drugs (*continued*).

may relapse in a leisurely and completely unpredictable rate over months and even years. There are only a few patients who relapse so rapidly that a minimum maintenance dosage can actually be determined easily.

In recent years, clinicians working with intermittent antipsychotic medication strategies in chronic schizophrenic patients aver that identifying the individual patient's unique signs of impending relapse (e.g., poor sleep, pacing, special fears or worries) can enable the treating psychiatrist to reinstitute antipsychotic medication rapidly and thus avert a full psychotic episode (Carpenter and Heinrichs 1983; Herz et al. 1982). Enlisting both patient and family to identify such early warning signs and symptoms and to watch for their reemergence is beneficial. This technique can be applied as well to gradual dose-tapering strategies. Careful patient monitoring by both caretakers and mental health professionals is necessary for this strategy to work well.

Although the available drugs differ in their side effects, on average and—less predictably—in individual patients, there are no obvious overall differences between the standard antipsychotic drugs in clinical efficacy in particular types of schizophrenic patients or in stages of illness on which to base the choice of a particular drug. The clinician can guess that an anxious, excited, acutely psychotic patient may respond better to a sedative drug like chlorpromazine, or the clinician can guess that a less sedative but less hypotensive drug like haloperidol might be better because relatively larger doses are likely to be better tolerated. Either choice is acceptable.

There is a small series of studies by Van Putten (1978) that show that if the first dose of an antipsychotic is judged even slightly helpful by a patient, that patient will have a good response to the drug over a 4-week trial, whereas if the first dose is unpleasant because of oversedation or early signs of akathisia, the patient will do badly during a 4-week trial even if antiparkinsonian drugs and dosage adjustment are used to their best advantage. (It may be—although no one has tried such an irregular approach—that one should give acutely ill patients a different drug every day until one is found that the patient does not dislike.) The inverse of this is to take good drug histories, whenever possible, and to avoid drugs that the patient remembers to have been unpleasant.

The drugs *do* differ in the dosages and formulations in which they are available. Thioridazine, chlorprothixene, pimozide, and clozapine are not available in parenteral forms. Generic, and therefore less expensive, forms are now available for chlorpromazine, trifluoperazine, and thioridazine, and the patent on several others including haloperidol will be expiring shortly. So far, there is no evidence that generic forms are significantly different from the original product, but some patients will strongly prefer the old standby.

Haloperidol may have a special tactical advantage in having a tasteless, colorless elixir, whereas the chlorpromazine and thioridazine elixirs, at least, taste very medicinal. A list of available dosages and formulations is given in Table 4-1. The cost per 100 tablets is given in the Appendix.

Only fluphenazine and haloperidol are available in long-acting depot preparations in the United States. A number of other depot drugs (fluspiriline, flupentixol, perphenazine) plus an oral tablet (penfluridol), which lasts a week, are available in Europe and, in some cases, Canada. Depot fluphenazine is available both as the enanthate and the decanoate, but there is no clear evidence that these are notably different from each other. Haloperidol is available as the decanoate only.

Since one of the main reasons antipsychotics do not work is because patients dislike them and refuse to take them, depot fluphenazine has the great advantage that a known amount of drug is administered reliably and that the staff is immediately aware when an injection is missed. Several controlled studies have failed, however, to show that depot fluphenazine is any more effective than oral fluphenazine in averting psychotic relapse in aftercare patients. Our interpretation of these counterintuitive data is that research studies with dedicated nurses and excellent outreach and weekly medication monitoring, with all patients getting both pills and injections, provide an excellent but unreal level of aftercare that ensures both pill and injection taking. In more typical understaffed aftercare programs, depot fluphenazine injections will most likely be much easier to monitor and will be better monitored than pill taking. More "naturalistic" studies would have likely shown depot drug to be better at averting relapse, especially in patients with a history of noncompliance. It is not uncommon to find that patients who have repeatedly stopped taking oral antipsychotic medication after hospital discharge and have vociferously objected to taking medication will cooperate faithfully with a depot neuroleptic regimen, presenting themselves for the injection on time month after month. The reasons for this improved compliance are unclear. One possibility is that patients who stop oral antipsychotic medications feel "better" in a few days as the side effects wear off. Some patients even become transiently euphoric before going on to become grossly psychotic. Stopping oral medication may therefore be rein- . forcing to the patient, whereas delaying depot injections is not.

The next issue is the comparative potencies of the various available antipsychotics. Several experts have tried their hand at determining this. Our version is in Table 4-2.

One last general comment about antipsychotics is in order. Although we can think of very few reasons for using two antipsychotics concurrently, there is no evidence that such a practice would be toxic or hazardous to the patient. Polypharmacy is generally frowned upon, and the use of two antipsychotics together requires a clinical justification. The only one that comes readily to mind is the use of a sedative, low-potency antipsychotic at bedtime and a high-potency antipsychotic during the day in the rare patient who has insomnia on the high-potency drug alone but is oversedated if a low-potency drug is used by itself to control psychopathology. Also, many neuroleptics lack a parenteral formulation; a patient receiving oral thioridazine and requiring a parenteral as needed will inevitably receive a second neuroleptic.

THERAPY

Early Treatment and Crisis Intervention

Over the past few years, a great deal has been written and several small to medium-sized double-blind studies have been carried out to determine how best to medicate acutely psychotic, anxious, delusional, hallucinating, angry, bizarre

Table 4-2.   Antipsychotic drug potency

Generic name	Brand name	Chlorpromazine equivalence
acetophenazine	Tindal	4.25
chlorpromazine	Thorazine	1.00
chlorprothixene	Taractan	2.25
clozapine	Clozaril	1.65
fluphenazine HCl	Prolixin	85.00
fluphenazine decanoate	Prolixin Decanoate	1 cc/month = 400 mg/day
haloperidol	Haldol	62.50
loxapine	Loxitane	6.65
mesoridazine	Serentil	1.80
molindone	Moban	10.00
perphenazine	Trilafon	11.25
piperacetazine	Quide	9.50
prochlorperazine	Compazine	7.00
reserpine	Serpasil	66.70
thioridazine	Mellaril	1.00
thiothixene	Navane	19.20
trifluoperazine	Stelazine	35.70
triflupromazine	Vesprin	3.50

patients with presumptive schizophrenia or schizophreniform or manic conditions who present in emergency rooms or are newly admitted to psychiatric wards. There are strong proponents of intensive megadose regimens such as "rapid neuroleptization," in which dosages on the order of 10 mg of haloperidol every hour or 5 mg every half hour or even a single 30-mg loading dose is given until the patient becomes calm. Probably any of the high-potency drugs could be used, although only haloperidol, fluphenazine, loxapine, and thiothixene have been studied systematically. Chlorpromazine was previously prescribed in such situations, but repeated dosages of 50 mg intramuscularly will cause patients to be oversedated and seriously hypotensive, whereas very large repeated doses of the high-potency drugs noted above are better tolerated (except for the side effects of dystonia and akathisia).

Droperidol, marketed only for use in anesthesia, may be the most rapidly effective drug given parenterally. It is quite sedative. There are a few reports from emergency psychiatric services describing excellent results with parenteral droperidol as the main initial medication for disturbed, excited psychotic patients. There is one controlled study showing that 5 mg of droperidol was better than 5 mg of haloperidol parenterally in terms of the proportion of patients requiring additional medication one half hour later. Although droperidol has been described as being effective in dosages of 5–20 mg intramuscularly or intravenously, the drug is not FDA-approved for psychiatric conditions, only for use in anesthesia. Clinicians wishing to use it would be well advised to use 2.5–5 mg of droperidol intramuscularly and to use it only where adequate medical backup (intubation, oxygen, etc.) is available. It is used occasionally with fair success at McLean Hospital in persistently disturbed and violent patients. Patients receiving droperidol often sleep longer and are quieter than patients receiving other parenteral neuroleptics, lorazepam, or amobarbital sodium. So far we have had no problems with its use.

It is easy to see why the clinician or ward or crisis unit staff confronted by a strikingly psychotic patient might wish to pull out all the stops in an attempt to achieve rapid reduction in psychosis. Unfortunately, the data from controlled studies to date show only that a very high dose (e.g., 100 mg of haloperidol or 200 mg of fluphenazine per day) has no advantage over a low dose, even in the first few hours of treatment. It is not even clear that intramuscular medication acts more rapidly than oral medication, and it is even possible, though unproven, that 2 mg of lorazepam given intramuscularly may produce more rapid calming in such situations. (See reviews by both Ayd [1985] and Cole [1982].)

A conservative but effective approach is to give a moderate dose of an antipsychotic (e.g., 5 mg of haloperidol, 25 mg of loxapine, 2 mg of fluphenazine, or even 50 mg of chlorpromazine) and wait, adding a benzodiazepine if the patient continues to be overexcited after an hour or two. Intramuscular medication can be given if the patient is a danger to self or others, but oral medication can often be used. Liquid medication is preferable because patients may cheek tablets or capsules and avoid swallowing them. The patient should be started on a sensible, modest daily dose of an antipsychotic as indicated.

In situations of rampaging, uncontrollable, dangerous psychosis in patients who have to be held in open, nonpsychiatric facilities, restraint and more frequent larger doses may be unavoidable, but one may well be treating the situation rather than the patient. Droperidol intramuscularly at 2.5 mg (or 5 mg in large, very violent patients) may have an advantage over other parenteral antipsychotics because of its rapid onset of action and prolonged sedative effect (see above). It is possible that the patients who have been enrolled in double-blind acute studies differ from those who are claimed to require crash, high-dose neuroleptization, but it is best to keep doses as low as possible in all situations.

Early Inpatient Treatment

There is no evidence that dosages higher than 15 mg of haloperidol or 400 mg of chlorpromazine a day or the equivalent are any more effective during the first few weeks of treatment than the above, reasonably standard low doses. Probably doses as low as 4 mg of haloperidol, 7 mg of fluphenazine, or 200 mg of thioridazine are adequate. In fact, a recent unpublished study (by McEvoy at Pittsburgh) using the detection of minimal arm cogwheeling as an indicator that a neuroleptic threshold had been reached (well short of major neurological side effects) found the average threshold dose of haloperidol to be 3.8 mg a day and found good improvement rates over a 6-week trial.

As noted above, schizophrenic patients improve relatively

slowly, showing some change in the first week of treatment with further improvement up to the sixth week. This improvement can occur over a wide range of dosages. Acute controlled drug studies generally fail to find an antipsychotic dose so low that improvement does not occur, while very high doses are *less* effective than lower dosages. So far, we know of no acute inpatient study that has found a dose too low to be effective.

The psychiatrist faced with a disturbed patient and a concerned or even frightened ward staff who ordinarily use high neuroleptic dosages and frequent prn medication may be hard put to keep to a low, sensible, steady dosage regimen, but we strongly believe that the latter alternative is best. Again, the use of oral and parenteral benzodiazepines such as lorazepam may be more useful than giving higher dosages of neuroleptic, and they may provide more benefit to both patient and staff.

Picking the "right" drug for the patient may not be possible, and the actual drug used may often be irrelevant, all available neuroleptics being essentially equivalent in average efficacy. Nevertheless, it is well worth getting a detailed drug history from patients, family, and past physicians for patients with prior antipsychotic therapy. The point is to find out which drugs the patient has received and responded to—or those the patient has had bad reactions to or disliked actively—and to try to pick a drug that the patient will respond to.

Thioridazine should probably be avoided in sexually active younger males because of its sexual side effects, unless these patients have had akathisia or dystonia on higher-potency drugs. We tend to use haloperidol, trifluoperazine, thiothixene, and loxapine more than other drugs for no documentable reason other than general personal preference. We have recently become impressed by the number of acutely psychotic patients who show little response to relatively high dosages of perphenazine and have been using the drug less often in manic and schizophrenic patients. Molindone might be preferred in overweight patients because of its tendency to promote modest weight loss. As noted in Chapter 1, it is sensible to stick with a few drugs so that one becomes familiar with their dosages and idiosyncracies. The only other consideration is that recurrently or chronically relapsing psychotic patients might be started on oral fluphenazine or oral haloperidol to see if it is well tolerated as an intermediate step toward shifting the patient to the depot preparation. Patients with insomnia that is not responsive to high-potency, low-dose neuroleptics could be shifted to chlorpromazine or chlorprothixene (100–300 mg) at bedtime for greater hypnotic effect. If a patient actively dislikes the first few doses of a particular antipsychotic, it seems reasonable to try one or two others to see if the patient will feel less bad and cooperate more.

In the early days of treatment, liquid medication is preferable to ensure ingestion, and doses should probably be divided, with lower doses given two or three times a day and a higher dose at bedtime. There is no clear evidence that this is any more effective than once-a-day or twice-a-day regimens, but it may make treatment induction smoother.

Similarly, prn dosages in agitated patients have no proven efficacy but are often appreciated by ward staff and sometimes by patients, since they give the impression that the crisis is being managed. Perhaps prn prescription of a benzodiazepine—lorazepam at 1 or 2 mg or diazepam at 5 mg—would, in fact, give more symptomatic relief, and parenteral sodium amobarbital or lorazepam may be more effective in quieting a wildly excited patient who is already receiving antipsychotics on a regular basis.

Some patients may become oversedated as their symptoms improve. If this occurs, the neuroleptic dose should be adjusted downward.

If a patient does not improve on an adequate dose of an antipsychotic, there are several choices available, although the reasons for selecting a specific one remain obscure. A different antipsychotic drug can be tried, of course. However, in the absence of undesirable side effects, it is always difficult to be sure whether a shift to a different drug at a more or less equivalent dose will do better than continuing the original drug for a longer period. Pragmatically, 2 weeks without response in a markedly psychotic patient and 5–6 weeks in a patient with milder symptoms or with detectable but quite inadequate improvement generally forces the clinician to make a change or to add a different class of drug such as lithium. Again, the choice of the second drug is more clearly determined by the patient's past untoward reactions to specific neuroleptics than by any rational strategy based on the patient's specific pattern of psychopathology. There are, however, limited data suggesting chlorpromazine may be worth trying in badly disorganized, markedly thought-disordered patients, and loxapine may be preferred in paranoid schizophrenia (Bishop et al. 1977). Shifting chemical class sounds rational, but no one really knows whether fluphenazine resembles, say, perphenazine more than haloperidol or molindone. Some clinicians end up selecting the last drug that worked for them in a similar treatment-resistant patient.

Since patients who are failing to respond have usually already been tried on higher dosages of the original antipsychotic without benefit, it is better to use the time of change to see if a substantially lower equivalent dose of the new drug will be any better. Again, if the second drug is well tolerated, it should be continued for several weeks. The only situation in which changing drugs can be dramatic is a shift to parenteral or depot medication in a patient who has not actually been taking his or her oral medication. As Donald Klein once said, "The first thing to do when a drug isn't working is to make sure the patient is actually taking it!"

When the patient is not improving and is taking a substantial dose of an antipsychotic, it is possible that akinesia, akathisia, or confusion due to the anticholinergic effects of antiparkinsonian drugs may be responsible. One can decrease

the dose rapidly to that equivalent to 400 mg of chlorpromazine a day and expect some rebound agitation followed,
sometimes, by significant improvement.

It is too early to be certain whether neuroleptic plasma
levels will be of major value in titrating dose, but there are
enough suggestions of the existence of a therapeutic window
with some antipsychotics that plasma levels could be tried
cautiously in patients who do not improve. "Therapeutic"
ranges really do not exist, but laboratories can provide
commonly observed blood level ranges. If a patient's blood
level (12 hours after an oral dose or a week after a depot
injection) is either very high or almost undetectable, then
appropriate changes can be tried. If the patient is already on
a very high dose of a neuroleptic and the laboratory finds
almost none in the blood, one should change drugs (or
laboratories) or double-check on compliance. We worry about
escalating neuroleptics to huge dosages on laboratory data
alone unless one has access to an outstandingly competent
laboratory.

At this time, the best evidence for rational relationships
between plasma levels and clinical response exists for haloperidol. There may even be a curvilinear relationship such
that levels below 4 ng/ml or above 26 ng/ml are associated
with poorer clinical response than levels within this 4–26
ng/ml "window." However, not all studies agree, and clinicians wishing to use this guideline must determine for
themselves whether the levels are useful. The clinically con-
vincing event occurs when a nonresponding patient improves
when a level outside the window is adjusted to fall within it.

In patients who appear not to be responding to treatment,
careful reevaluation of the patient for overt and covert side
effects is necessary. Addition (or removal) of antiparkinsonian
drugs or other medications designed to alleviate specific side
effects or shifting to another neuroleptic may be helpful.
Even moving the whole dose to bedtime may help by
decreasing daytime sedation or inertia. Reconsidering diag-

nosis is also helpful. Some patients initially assumed to be schizophrenic may turn out to fit psychotic depression or atypical mania better, and the addition of an antidepressant or lithium may be positively indicated.

Some treatment-resistant DSM-III-R schizophrenic patients with little or nothing in the way of affective symptoms can improve with the addition of lithium to an antipsychotic, although this rarely results in a full remission. Perhaps anxious, dysphoric patients are more likely to benefit. If a patient is unremittingly and seriously psychotic and quite probably either worse or no better on antipsychotic drugs, he or she needs to be tried off all antipsychotics to make sure that he or she is not made worse by them. Moreover, their use, in the face of little apparent response, needs to be justified because of the risk of dyskinesia.

This advice is remarkably hard to implement in many clinical situations, which is a great pity. It should also be remembered that electroconvulsive therapy *is* effective in catatonic excitements and is often helpful, at least to terminate an episode, in drug-resistant schizophrenic patients. It is also worth doing toxic urine screens and determining blood phencyclidine levels to make sure the patient is not continuing to take illicit drugs even while in the hospital.

Maintenance Drug Therapy

There is no evidence as to how long to keep a patient who has recovered from a first psychotic episode on neuroleptic therapy. Probably stopping the drug 2 days after the patient appears much better will lead to a return of psychosis, whereas after 3 months many patients, perhaps 85%, might tolerate 3 weeks off medication without relapsing. At some point, the drug action seems to shift from being directly antipsychotic to preventing relapse. In principle, and generally in practice, schizophrenic patients reach a stable level of remission, often with residual psychotic symptoms that do not, then, improve with increased medication and even may not worsen when the drug is stopped; in fact, some patients feel "better," with more alertness and energy, off medication. However, the risk of relapse is a good deal greater off medication. Perhaps one-fifth of all patients stabilized on antipsychotic medication will show signs of increasing psychosis as the drug is being tapered—good evidence that the medication is necessary.

To return to the first-episode patient in full remission, prolonged antipsychotic treatment is not indicated, but it seems sensible to keep the patient on a very gradually decreasing dose of the drug on which he or she improved for at least 3 months after discharge or from the point of marked improvement. If the patient will be under predictable stress in the next 6–9 months (e.g., completing school, starting a new job, getting divorced), we favor continuing the neuroleptic until that stress point is well past and the patient is generally coping adequately.

For patients with a history of two or more psychotic episodes that appear to come on after they have been taken or have taken themselves off antipsychotics, maintenance antipsychotic therapy is indicated.

This issue is under serious review, however, and systematic large-scale studies are under way that may challenge our old beliefs. Kane's work suggests that as little as about 2.5 mg (0.1 ml) of fluphenazine decanoate every 2 weeks (actually 10% of the fluphenazine decanoate dose on which the patient has been clinically stable) is more effective than placebo in preventing relapse though less effective than the full (100%) dose (Kane et al. 1983). The 10% dose illustrates current risk-benefit problems; the patients on this dose appear to feel better and function a bit better and are judged better by their families than patients on the 100% dose and also develop fewer dyskinetic movements but relapse into psychosis more! Is this "better" or "worse" overall? Several studies suggest that a 20% dose (e.g., about 5 mg every 2 weeks) is as effective as the full dose at preventing relapse for the first year only; in the second year, the group on the 20% dose had more relapses than the group on the full dose.

The other option, espoused by both Carpenter and Herz, is that patients with recurring schizophrenic relapses should be followed every 2–4 weeks but should receive drug therapy only when and if they show symptoms of impending relapse. This approach requires careful work with the patient, family, and caretakers to identify signs and symptoms of impending relapse unique to each patient so that medication can be restarted before full psychosis is manifest and hospitalization mandatory. It is still unclear whether this option will be better or worse in terms of long-term outcome or short-term social adjustment or occurrence of tardive dyskinesia than the other two options. Preliminary (unpublished) results from two studies indicate that steady medication is more effective than intermittent therapy in preventing relapse.

At the moment, we favor stabilizing chronic relapsing schizophrenic patients in the community for 3–6 months, then tapering the dose very slowly over 6–9 months to about 50% of the initial therapeutic dose, increasing the dose if psychotic or dysphoric symptoms reemerge.

Other problems in maintenance antipsychotic therapy are evident. First, maintenance only averts relapse in about half of the patients on that regimen. Second, it is often very hard to determine whether the patient relapsed because of stopping the antipsychotic medication or whether the patient stopped the medication because he or she began to relapse. Third, as tardive dyskinesia gradually emerges, the clinician gets more and more uncomfortable about continuing medication. Fourth, many chronic schizophrenic patients well stabilized in the community get very rigid about their treatment, and get upset (and relapse) if their medication is changed. We recently had several long-term aftercare patients who had been on neuroleptics for over 5 years relapse with as little as a 40% decrease in their antipsychotic dose. In another study, investigators withdrew active medication in schizophrenic patients stable in the community for 5 years and found an 80% relapse rate over the following year, suggesting that low-dose maintenance drug therapy may be necessary for prolonged periods.

Maintenance antipsychotic therapy in nonschizophrenic patients is *not*, generally, a good idea at all. The risk of dyskinesia is real, and the burden is on the clinician to prove that maintenance therapy was, in fact, necessary and effective. This can, of course, sometimes be the case. Trials off medication to demonstrate continued need for it are not clearly indicated in recurring chronic schizophrenia but are really required to defend maintenance neuroleptic therapy in mental retardation, affective disorders, demented elderly patients, or patients with borderline or other personality disorders.

Use in Depression

In psychotic depression there is good evidence that perphenazine combined with amitriptyline is superior to either drug alone. There is no reason to believe that there is anything magical about this pair of drugs. Probably, any antidepressant plus any antipsychotic could work about as well. There is limited evidence that amoxapine alone can be useful in psychotic depression. Electroconvulsive therapy is undeniably effective in psychotic depression, perhaps more effective than tricyclic-neuroleptic combinations. The dosages of neuroleptics used in psychotic depression are often quite high (e.g., 48–72 mg of perphenazine); it is unclear whether such high dosages are necessary.

When antipsychotics are used in depression, the medical record should reflect the reasons clearly. When the drug is continued for several months, the risks of dyskinesia must be noted and the need for maintenance neuroleptic use strongly justified. Many malpractice suits for tardive dyskinesia involve depressed patients who develop dyskinesia on antipsychotics. Data from McLean Hospital suggest that unipolar depressed patients, psychotic or nonpsychotic, develop dyskinesia twice as early and on half the drug exposure of schizophrenic patients.

Of the available neuroleptics, only thioridazine is approved by the FDA for use in depression—moderate to marked depression with anxiety or agitation. There are occasional depressed patients who appear to be uniquely responsive to antipsychotics and fail to improve on more conventional antidepressants. Some clinicians add low doses of antipsychotics to standard antidepressants as adjuvants in an attempt to convert a nonresponding patient into a responder in much the same way that lithium or thyroid is used. There are no solid clinical studies supporting these practices, but they can be justified if the patient is kept on the antipsychotic only if he or she substantially benefits from it.

Use in Anxiety

Although very low doses of neuroleptics (25 mg of chlorpromazine, 0.5 mg of haloperidol, 2 mg of trifluoperazine, 2 mg of thiothixene) given two or three times a day or in equivalent amounts at bedtime to promote sleep are sometimes effective in generalized anxiety disorder, this regimen has not been extensively studied. As noted in Chapter 6, tricyclic antidepressants carry less risk and are probably at least as effective as antipsychotic drugs. Neuroleptics should only be used in anxiety states when more appropriate drugs fail.

Recent studies of the use of antipsychotics in patients with borderline personality disorder or schizotypal personality disorder show that they benefit from low-dose neuroleptic treatment. The available studies have covered a period of only a few months and have involved haloperidol, thiothixene, thioridazine, trifluoperazine, and depot flupentixol, one study per drug. A reasonable interpretation of all this is that antipsychotics have a stabilizing effect on irritability, mood lability, and impulsivity and decrease anxiety. They may have a use in the early stages of a more comprehensive treatment program for borderline patients. Prolonged antipsychotic treatment for over 6 months should not be undertaken unless the patient and doctor are clear that major benefit is continuing, because of the risk of dyskinesia. Again, documenting the reasons for neuroleptic use in the beginning and periodically later in treatment is mandatory.

Use in Organic States

Antipsychotics are widely used in agitated organic states such as delirium, senile dementia, and mental retardation with little evidence that they are really helpful. Sometimes they cause more harm through side effects than they do good, and their use is strictly empirical—valuable only if they help (see Chapter 12).

In conditions such as depression, anxiety, personality disorder, or organic brain syndromes where efficacy is not firmly established, other drug therapies or no drug therapy may be preferable.

The use of antipsychotics should *never* be routine, and their effects and their effectiveness for each particular patient should always be carefully monitored and documented.

SIDE EFFECTS

Sedation

Sedation, often accompanied by fatigue, can be useful early in treatment but a liability after the patient is improved. All antipsychotics can be sedative in some patients at some dose, but chlorpromazine is generally the most sedative. Its sedative effects are often judged very unpleasant by normal volunteers receiving even 25 mg or 50 mg of the drug in a single dose, but they are sometimes accepted or even welcomed by some psychotic or personality disorder patients. Thioridazine, chlorprothixene, and loxapine are also often relatively sedative, whereas the other high-potency antipsychotics are often less sedative or not at all so. In one acute dosage strategy, the antipsychotic dosage is gradually raised until the psychosis is controlled, at which point the patient will develop increased sedation, which then requires dosage reduction.

In chronic administration, sedation and fatigue overlap with akinesia, a side effect characterized by inertia, inactivity, and lack of spontaneous movement. Akinesia will often abate when an antiparkinsonian drug is added or, slowly, when the dose is lowered.

When antipsychotics are used as prn medication, it is likely that sedation is the main effect produced even though decrease in psychosis may be desired. As has been discussed, a benzodiazepine (e.g., 1 or 2 mg of lorazepam) may be more appropriate for this purpose. Unfortunately, the short- (or long-) term utility of prn medication of any sort, whether as a favor to the patient or as chemical restraint, has never been seriously studied.

Autonomic Side Effects

All antipsychotics can cause postural hypotension, but this is presumed to be more common and severe with the low-potency drugs, at least with chlorpromazine and thioridazine, and more dangerous in elderly or infirm patients.

Antipsychotics also have anticholinergic effects, most striking with thioridazine but also clear with chlorpromazine, mesoridazine, and trifluoperazine; they are also present but to a lesser degree with the other drugs. Dry mouth and nasal congestion can occur, as can visual blurring. When antipsychotics are combined with other anticholinergic drugs (antiparkinsonian or tricyclic antidepressant drugs), delirium or bowel stasis can occur. Constipation is a milder form of this effect.

Retrograde ejaculation is fairly common with thioridazine and can occur with other drugs in this class. This can progress to impotence. It is worth inquiring about sexual effects, since patients may be upset by them but hesitate to mention them spontaneously.

Endocrine Effects

The direct effect of antipsychotic drugs is an increase in blood prolactin levels. There is a large and complex literature on this, since prolactin levels have been proposed as an alternative to measuring antipsychotic blood level directly. Attempts to use prolactin level as a guide to adequate dosage in newly hospitalized patients have not been validated to date, but one study has suggested that aftercare patients with low prolactin levels are more likely to relapse than those with higher levels.

Hyperprolactinemia can cause breast enlargement and galactorrhea in both female and male patients and may play a role in the impotence in males and the amenorrhea in female patients seen occasionally with these drugs. Dopaminergic drugs such as amantadine (200–300 mg/day) or bromocriptine (7.5–15 mg/day) can be tried to reduce prolactin levels.

Weight gain, often quite excessive, can occur on all antipsychotic drugs. It is unclear whether this is a result of increased appetite or decreased activity. Molindone is believed to be less likely to cause weight gain and even may cause modest weight loss, again for unknown reasons. Although all antipsychotics except thioridazine are good antiemetics, nausea and vomiting are sometimes seen as side effects for reasons not yet determined.

Skin and Eye Complications

A variety of allergic skin rashes can occur with antipsychotics as with all other drugs, but are more common with chlorpromazine.

Chlorpromazine on prolonged high-dose administration can cause pigmentation of areas exposed to light and can cause pigment deposits in the eye, chiefly in the back of the cornea and the front of the lens. These almost never affect vision and do not require regular slit lamp examinations, but patients showing an opaque pupil when a light is shone into the eye should have an ophthalmological evaluation. These deposits probably only occur with chlorpromazine but could conceivably occur with other drugs.

Retinal pigmentation occurs only with thioridazine (never reported, so far, with thioridazine's metabolite mesoridazine), and its serious and irreversible effect on vision requires that thioridazine dosage be kept at or below 800 mg a day.

Chlorpromazine often causes skin photosensitivity manifested as a severe sunburn in exposed skin areas after relatively brief (30–60 minutes) exposure to direct sunlight. Block-Out or an equivalent sunscreen containing para-aminobenzoic acid (PABA), which screens out ultraviolet rays, will help avoid this effect. Other antipsychotics *may* cause photosensitivity, and patients are generally advised to wear sunscreens. Sun sensitivity can best be determined by cautious exposure to the sun in gradually increased durations. Many patients will prove to tolerate the sun normally. Chlorpromazine should be avoided in patients who are likely to spend long periods out-of-doors at work or for pleasure.

Patients on chlorpromazine for prolonged periods of time can develop a slate gray to purplish pigmentation of skin areas exposed to sunlight. This probably fades slowly once the drug is stopped.

Other or Rare Complications

Agranulocytosis has been associated with chlorpromazine and thioridazine and could presumably occur with other antipsychotics. Its incidence is low, perhaps 1 case in 5,000 patients treated. It usually comes on in the first 3 months of treatment. Monitoring for agranulocytosis does not require frequent or regular blood counts. However, patients developing a sore throat and fever in the first few months of therapy require an emergency blood count to rule out this rare but serious complication. Leukopenias in the 3,000–4,000 range also occur and are not generally serious, whereas agranulocytosis, often defined as a white blood cell count of less than 2,000 cells/m^3 with less than 500 cells/m^3 of polymorphonuclear leukocytes, is very serious and requires immediate medical attention by a hematologist. Needless to say, clinicians should seriously consider stopping a drug if the white blood cell count is less than 3,000 cells/m^3.

A form of allergic obstructive hepatitis was reported relatively frequently in the early days of chlorpromazine use with an incidence of 2–3%, but this has been much more rarely encountered in recent years. Even when it occurred it was a relatively mild transient disorder that did not lead to hepatic necrosis or permanent liver damage. Liver problems occur so rarely with other antipsychotics as to make one believe that the occasionally abnormal liver function tests seen in patients on these drugs are due to some intercurrent, unrelated event or drug. Such abnormalities, unless progressive and severe, are not a reason for discontinuing an effective antipsychotic in a patient who needs the drug, although internists tend to blame the antipsychotic without an adequate basis when abnormal liver function tests are observed.

Seizures can also occur in patients treated with antipsychotics. Only promazine (no longer used) caused them with any frequency. We know of no good data available on the comparative effects of these drugs on seizure threshold but tend to suspect loxapine and chlorpromazine as being involved in the rare neuroleptic-related seizures seen at McLean Hospital and presume that the high-potency drugs are less likely to cause seizures. Certainly, patients with known epilepsy who are receiving anticonvulsants often receive antipsychotics without any obvious effect on seizure frequency.

Sudden death has been associated with antipsychotic use in healthy young adults. The mechanisms suggested include ventricular fibrillation and aspiration of food or of vomitus during a grand mal seizure, but no clear etiology is proven. Since such deaths occurred in young psychiatric patients before antipsychotic drugs were discovered, its connection with medication remains tenuous. Over the last 30 years we have heard of more sudden deaths on thioridazine (four) than on any other neuroleptic, but even these are so very rare as to make suspicion unwarranted.

Neurological Side Effects

Although dopamine blockade in the striatum is the most popular mechanism invoked for all neurological side effects from antipsychotic drugs and anticholinergic antiparkinsonian drugs are the conventional remedy, the presumed cholinergic-dopaminergic imbalance is probably only a partial explanation.

Dystonia. The earliest side effect, dystonia, often manifested by tonic muscle spasm in the tongue, jaw, and neck, usually occurs in the first few hours or days on an antipsychotic. It can present as a very frightening opisthotonos of the whole body with extensor rigidity or as only mild tongue stiffness. In one small study dystonia appeared as neuroleptic blood levels were dropping, not rising, making one wonder whether it might be a rebound effect as dopamine blockade is waning. In any event, it can be fairly effectively averted by prophylactic antiparkinsonian usage (Table 4-3) and rarely occurs with thioridazine. It is more common in younger males but can occur in either sex at any age. Once present, it can be rapidly relieved by intravenous antiparkinsonian drugs (only diphen-hydramine and biperiden are readily available for parenteral use) or, less rapidly, by intramuscular medication. However, such diverse drugs as diazepam, amobarbital, and caffeine sodium benzoate and even hypnosis have been said to relieve it as well.

Once the dystonia has resolved and the patient is protected by oral antiparkinsonian medication, the offending antipsy-chotic can be continued without recurrence of the dystonia, but patients often feel less apprehensive if a different anti-psychotic drug is substituted. Some patients on depot flu-phenazine will develop recurrences of dystonia with succeed-ing injections.

Oculogyric crises, manifested by forced eye rotation, usu-ally upward, are conventionally classified with the dystonias but can occur, even recur fairly frequently, later in treatment when more conventional dystonia is rare.

Pseudoparkinsonism.   Some time in the early stages of treat-ment, usually between 5 days and 4 weeks, the patient can develop signs of parkinsonism. In contrast to idiopathic Parkinson's disease, pill-rolling tremor is very rare, but muscle stiffness, cogwheel rigidity, stooped posture, masklike facies, and even drooling are quite common. Micrographia occurs and can help differentiate antipsychotic tremor from lithium tremor.

Patients rarely develop such severe parkinsonian rigidity as to be incapacitated or even immobilized. When they do, such patients are sometimes misdiagnosed as having cata-tonia. Patients with such severe rigidity do not respond readily to even massive doses of antiparkinsonian drugs; the condition may require as long as 2 weeks to clear after the antipsychotic drug is stopped.

Table 4-3. Antiparkinsonian drugs

Generic name	Brand name	Formulations	Dosage ranges (mg/day)
Primarily anticholinergic			
benztropine	Cogentin*	Tablet: 1, 2 mg Parenteral: 1 mg/ml (2-ml ampule)	2–6
biperiden	Akineton	Tablet: 2 mg Parenteral: 5 mg/ml (1-ml ampule)	2–8
diphenhydramine	Benadryl*	Capsule: 25, 50 mg Elixir: 12.5 mg/5 ml (4-oz, 16-oz bottle) Parenteral: 10 mg/ml (10-ml, 30-ml vial), 1-ml ampule	50–300
ethopropazine	Parsidol	Tablet: 10, 50 mg	100–400
procyclidine	Kemadrin	Tablet: 5 mg	10–20
trihexyphenidyl	Artane*	Tablet: 2, 5 mg Sequels: 5-mg capsule	4–15
Dopaminergic			
amantadine	Symmetrel*	Capsule: 100 mg Syrup: 50 mg/5 ml (16-oz bottle)	100–300

* Available in generic form.

Milder degrees of pseudoparkinsonism are often seen for prolonged periods in patients on long-term maintenance medication and can contribute to passive inactivity in such patients.

Akinesia—reduction in spontaneous or voluntary movement—can be seen in patients on maintenance antipsychotic medication in the absence of signs of parkinsonism; regular coarse tremor can also be seen alone without any other parkinsonian signs. Both conditions respond either to antiparkinsonian drugs or reduction in neuroleptic dose.

Akathisia.   This inner-driven restlessness caused by antipsychotics is the least understood and most troublesome of their neurological side effects. It ranges from an unpleasant subjective feeling of muscular discomfort to an agitated, desperate, markedly dysphoric pacing with hand-wringing and weeping. In between these extremes, patients will find themselves unable to sit still for long, having to stand up and move about or continually shift their position. Akathisia is sometimes mistaken for psychotic agitation and treated inappropriately by an increase in antipsychotic dose. It can be experienced even after the first dose of a neuroleptic but can become a clinical problem at any time in the first few weeks on medication. It occurs with thioridazine as well as with the more potent drugs. It is less responsive to antiparkinsonian drugs than other neurological side effects and is the bane of maintenance medication, being a common basis for patients refusing to stay on such a regimen. Recent studies suggest that propranolol in doses from 30 to 120 mg a day sometimes suppresses akathisia when neither antiparkinsonian drugs nor benzodiazepines such as lorazepam work. Its efficacy casts some doubt on dopamine blockade being the mechanism underlying akathisia.

Regular rhythmic leg jiggling up and down, or less commonly to and fro, is often seen in patients treated with antipsychotics and is probably, but not certainly, a variant of akathisia, although some consider it a form of tremor. Patients with this phenomenon are often unaware of it or not bothered by it. The best basis for differential diagnosis of akathisia is to ask the patient whether the restlessness is a "muscle" feeling or a "head" feeling—the former being akathisia and the latter, anxiety. In case of doubt, it is safer to assume akathisia exists since overdosage with neuroleptics is vastly more common than underdosage.

The drug therapy of akathisia often requires polypharmacy. Antiparkinsonian drugs, beta-blockers, and benzodiazepines all can be helpful in some patients but more than one of these agents may be required. Lowering the antipsychotic dosage should also be considered.

Use of Antiparkinsonian Drugs

For decades there have been impassioned arguments pro and con about the prophylactic use of antiparkinsonian drugs. Many senior clinicians claim that patient drug acceptance is enhanced and unpleasant side effects are averted by routine antiparkinsonian administration to all patients being started (or restarted) on antipsychotic drugs. Others, however, assert that two drugs (an antipsychotic drug plus an antiparkinsonian drug) can be more toxic than an antipsychotic alone and that an antiparkinsonian drug should only be added when neurological side effects appear. Personally, we believe there is enough evidence that antiparkinsonian drugs avert neurological side effects to use them routinely in most acutely psychotic patients under age 45 being started on a neuroleptic unless their anticholinergic side effects are contraindicated. In the less common situation in which very low dosage, cautious trials on antipsychotics (e.g., 1–3 mg of haloperidol a day) are undertaken, prophylactic antiparkinsonian drugs are unnecessary. If routine antiparkinsonian medication is not used prophylactically in acute patients, prn orders for such patients should be written.

After 4 weeks to 6 months of long-term maintenance antipsychotic therapy, the antiparkinsonian drugs can be shifted to prn or withdrawn. A few patients (approximately 15%) will redevelop clear neurological side effects and even more (approximately 30%) will feel "better"—less anxious or depressed or inert—on continued antiparkinsonian drugs. Some patients with chronic schizophrenia are delighted to stop their neuroleptic but demand to continue their antiparkinsonian drug (Wojcik 1979). Very rarely, patients use trihexyphenidyl or other antiparkinsonians to get "high," but far more patients do better on these drugs than off them.

There are rare patients who develop anticholinergic deliria or intestinal stasis on antiparkinsonian drugs; dry mouth and blurred vision are more common side effects. Dosage ranges of the available antiparkinsonian drugs are given in Table 4-3. Probably, if blood level determinations of either the drug itself or of anticholinergic levels by radioreceptor assay were generally available, dosage might be adjusted more rationally. At present, if a patient has neither relief of neurological side effects nor dry mouth, a cautious increase in dose—even over the maximum recommended in PDR—can be considered, although decreasing the neuroleptic dose may be even more rational.

Most of the antiparkinsonian drugs are assumed to work by their anticholinergic effects and are probably equivalent to one another, although we have seen rare syndromes that respond uniquely to the anticholinergic antihistamine diphenhydramine or to ethopropazine. No controlled comparative studies of these drugs exist to guide the clinician. Probably diphenhydramine is more sedative, trihexyphenidyl slightly more stimulating, and biperiden more neutral in this dimension.

Amantadine, which is presumed to work as a dopamine agonist, can be used at dosages of 200–300 mg a day. It is probably as effective as the anticholinergic antiparkinsonian drugs but has no proven advantages. Tolerance to its antiparkinsonian effects may also be more of a problem. However, it may be useful in galactorrhea by reducing blood prolactin levels. Although one might expect a dopamine agonist to be stimulant, patients sometimes find amantadine to be sedative.

Bromocriptine, another dopamine agonist, is available for prescription use and has been studied extensively in idiopathic Parkinson's disease. It may well prove useful in drug-induced pseudoparkinsonism and probably does not aggravate psychosis in patients on a stable neuroleptic dosage.

L-Dopa has not been systematically studied in pseudoparkinsonism. It probably works too slowly and can sometimes aggravate psychosis. The standard antiparkinsonian drugs generally have no obvious effect on the psychosis; the few controlled studies comparing antipsychotic drugs with and without added antiparkinsonian agents are equivocal.

Anticholinergic effects of the antiparkinsonian drugs can cause cognitive impairment in normal subjects and in schizophrenic patients. The magnitude and clinical importance of this effect is unclear but it is possible that mild memory problems caused by anticholinergic drug effects might well be missed in patients who were already cognitively impaired or sedated.

TARDIVE DYSKINESIA

Some patients exposed to antipsychotic drugs develop abnormal, involuntary, irregular, choreiform and/or athetoid movements. These most commonly include tongue overactivity—darting, writhing, twisting, or repeated protrusions—and finger movements—choreiform or hand clenching. Chewing or lateral jaw movements, lip puckering, facial grimacing, torticollis or retrocollis, trunk twisting, pelvic thrusting, respiratory grunting, athetoid arm and shoulder movements, or a variety of toe, ankle, and leg movements all occur in a variety of combinations. These are hard to distinguish, at times, from schizophrenic mannerisms and essentially impossible to distinguish on phenomenology alone from other, rarer causes of dyskinesia. Patients with typical movements of the sort described above are still referred to as having tardive dyskinesia. Those with major dystonic athetoid movements and sustained postures of the face, neck, arms, or trunk are referred to as having tardive dystonia, often a more severe and more incapacitating condition. Athetoid dystonic movements often coexist with the more typical tongue and lip movements of tardive dyskinesia. Tardive dystonia is more likely to be ameliorated by antiparkinsonian drugs than is conventional tardive dyskinesia. Tardive akathisia, a syndrome of forced motor restlessness persisting long after antipsychotic drugs have been stopped, can also occur. It is even less common than tardive dystonia.

The severity of tardive dyskinesia ranges from minimal tongue restlessness and finger movements to gross, incapacitating disfiguring movements. Most identifiable cases are mild and not noticed by either the patient or the family or are passed off as minor tics or restlessness by both. Even clearly visible dyskinesias are often of little real consequence, but about 3% of cases are sufficiently severe to cause social or functional problems. Most patients and families seen in the Tardive Dyskinesia Clinic at McLean Hospital are much more concerned about the possible ultimate consequences of currently very mild dyskinesia than about the minor movements the patient is showing at the time of consultation.

It is currently impossible to predict which patients will develop dyskinesia, early or late, mild or severe. However, the best available data suggest a rate of development of dyskinesia of about 2–4% per year over the first 7 years of exposure and that elderly women and patients with affective disorders may be at the greatest risk (Gardos and Casey 1984). In chronically institutionalized psychotic patients, dyskinesia prevalence rates are often on the order of 50–60%.

At the extremes, a few patients develop persistent dyskinesia after only a few weeks of exposure to antipsychotics, but up to 6 months on antipsychotics is generally considered safe. In our experience, about one-half the patients who develop overt dyskinesia do so on stable maintenance antipsychotic dosages, whereas about one-quarter first manifest dyskinesia when the neuroleptic is tapered or stopped (covert dyskinesia). Dyskinesia fades away in some patients when their antipsychotics are stopped weeks, months, or years later. Some patients lose their dyskinesia even on stable medication. There is a significant rate of occurrence of dyskinesia in individuals never exposed to neuroleptics, from 1 to 5%, increasing with advancing age so that not all dyskinesia in patients on neuroleptics is due to the drug. Unfortunately, no one can tell which cases are idiopathic. There are no strong, consistent treatment factors related to dyskinesia, either. Duration of antipsychotic treatment correlates more commonly with dyskinesia than does total dose. There is no clear evidence that any one antipsychotic is less commonly related to tardive dyskinesia development than any other.

Basic research data on dopamine receptor overproliferation caused by neuroleptics in laboratory animals have been used to claim that drugs such as thioridazine or molindone *should* be less likely to cause tardive dyskinesia than other antipsychotics, but we have seen a number of cases in patients only or almost only exposed to thioridazine and one case on molindone. In our experience, neither periods off neuroleptics nor extent of use of antiparkinsonian drugs seem generally related to tardive dyskinesia development, and lithium exposure does not seem to slow the emergence of dyskinesia. Thus, until some new, different, and safer antipsychotic emerges, there is no way to avoid tardive dyskinesia except to avoid using antipsychotics.

This means that the clinician must seriously consider the risks and benefits of extended treatment with antipsychotics in all patients likely to be kept on medication for longer than 6 months. This issue must be discussed with the patient and his or her family unless there are defensible clinical reasons for not doing so. Either way, everything should be documented in the patient's chart, and the process should be redone if signs of dyskinesia are noted. (See Chapter 1 for further discussion.)

To date, the available long-term (2- to 10-year) follow-up studies suggest that tardive dyskinesia is not generally a progressive disorder and can improve or vanish over time even on antipsychotics. In chronically psychotic patients, the best clinical decision is often to continue the antipsychotic, but this decision must be based on the available facts in each case.

There is no effective or standard treatment for tardive dyskinesia. Trying to slowly taper the antipsychotic dose is often recommended. Lithium is often added and the use of reserpine has its advocates. Also, a shift to a different antipsychotic is sometimes suggested. A recent smattering of small studies suggest that vitamin E (400 International Units bid) may gradually decrease dyskinesia. Diltiazem, a calcium channel blocker, at 30 mg po has been noted to decrease dyskinesia for a few hours. Neither approach has been thoroughly studied. Some, but not all, patients on clozapine show amelioration of dyskinesia either rapidly or slowly.

Unfortunately, tardive dyskinesia is a remarkably heterogeneous condition in terms of its response to drug therapies. Although the condition is often assumed to be due to dopaminergic overactivity and should therefore be suppressed by dopamine blocking agents and aggravated by anticholinergic antiparkinsonian drugs, some patients show exactly the opposite responses, and pseudoparkinsonism paradoxically often coexists with dyskinesia. Benzodiazepines often mildly alleviate dyskinetic movements. A vast range of other centrally active drugs have been tried and sometimes have helped. Luckily, most cases of dyskinesia are not serious enough to warrant special treatment.

Neuroleptic Malignant Syndrome

Neuroleptic malignant syndrome (NMS) is a potentially life-threatening complication of antipsychotic drug use. Estimates of its incidence vary from study to study, but a figure of 1% of all psychiatric admissions treated with neuroleptics seems reasonable, though rates as low as 0.07% and as high as 2.4% have been reported. Criteria for the diagnosis of NMS have fluctuated from article to article, but there is general agreement that all patients have hyperthermia, severe extrapyramidal signs, and autonomic dysfunction. Operational criteria currently in use at McLean Hospital are presented in Table 4-4, which provides a good description of the range of signs and symptoms that may be present.

Misdiagnosis can obviously occur when patients have fever caused by infection plus pseudoparkinsonism, but the severe muscle rigidity often seen in NMS is rare as an accompaniment of incidental infection. Serum creatinine kinase levels can be increased by intramuscular injections or violent physical struggling but rarely to a level as high as 1,000 IU/ml.

Neuroleptics can affect temperature-regulating brain centers and be associated with heatstroke, particularly in hot weather or in hot seclusion rooms, in the absence of other manifestations of NMS. A neuroleptic-induced catatonia, really a severe parkinsonian rigidity, can occur in the absence of fever.

NMS itself usually develops over 1–3 days in patients on antipsychotics. Many cases develop in the first week of drug treatment and most within the first month of treatment with antipsychotics. There is weak evidence that concomitant treatment with lithium may predispose patients to develop NMS. NMS has been observed with essentially all widely used neuroleptics, with thioridazine perhaps being under-represented. The dose of neuroleptic does not seem to be a major factor, although lower doses would seem likely to be

Table 4-4.   Operational criteria for diagnosis of neuroleptic malignant syndrome

The following three items all are required for a definite diagnosis:

1. **Hyperthermia:** Oral temperature of at least 38.0°C in the absence of another known etiology.
2. **Severe extrapyramidal effects** characterized by two or more of the following: lead-pipe muscle rigidity, pronounced cogwheeling, sialorrhea, oculogyric crisis, retrocollis, opisthotonos, trismus, dysphagia, choreiform movements, festinating gait, and flexor-extensor posturing.
3. **Autonomic dysfunction** characterized by two or more of the following: hypertension (at least 20-mm rise in diastolic pressure above baseline), tachycardia (at least 30 beats/minute), prominent diaphoresis, and incontinence.

In retrospective diagnosis, if one of these three items has not been specifically documented, a probable diagnosis is still permitted if the remaining two criteria are clearly met and the patient displays one of the following characteristic signs: clouded consciousness as evidenced by delirium, mutism, stupor, or coma; leukocytosis (more than 15,000 white blood cells/mm); and serum creatinine kinase level greater than 1,000 IU/ml.

safer. Depot neuroleptics do not seem more likely to cause NMS, but their prolonged duration of action will make the syndrome last far longer.

The best treatment is early identification, stopping neuroleptics, and, in moderate to severe cases, rapid transfer to a medical center. The dopamine agonist bromocriptine, at 5 mg every 4 hours, can often relieve muscle rigidity and reduce fever. Dantrolene is used in intensive care units to reduce the muscle spasm. Anticholinergic antiparkinsonian drugs are probably not helpful. Symptomatic treatment (e.g., cooling the body) is helpful.

The syndrome can recur after it appears to have come under control, so patients should be observed carefully for a month after the condition was first noted. Neuroleptics should be avoided during that period. We have successfully used electroconvulsive therapy in persistently manic patients who had recently experienced an episode of NMS.

In many, but not all, patients, neuroleptics can be restarted cautiously at much lower dosages without NMS recurring. It is not clear whether thioridazine is safer than one-quarter the dose of the original offending medication. It seems sensible to avoid depot antipsychotics in patients with a history of NMS.

NEWER ANTIPSYCHOTIC MEDICATIONS

Pimozide

Pimozide, a butyrophenone-like antipsychotic, is marketed in the United States only for the treatment of Tourette's syndrome but has been widely studied in Europe in the treatment of schizophrenia, where it has been reasonably effective.

Pimozide was prevented from being declared effective in the treatment of schizophrenia in this country, apparently because of the occurrence of some "cardiac events" in schizophrenic patients receiving the drug in dosages above 10 mg a day. There have been some, as far as we know, undocumented cardiac deaths associated with pimozide use in Canada. PDR notes that sudden unexpected deaths, presumably cardiac related, have occurred in patients on higher doses of pimozide. ECG monitoring is advised. The drug can prolong cardiac conduction time. Published European studies on the antipsychotic efficacy of pimozide have used dosages substantially higher than 10 mg a day and do not report any adverse cardiac effects.

Is pimozide worth using given the above uncertainty? Maybe. It is the purest dopamine-2 antagonist available and may be the polar opposite of clozapine, which is primarily a dopamine-1 blocker. Psychiatrists dealing with treatment-nonresponsive schizophrenic patients are often hard-pressed to find something different to try. Pimozide might possibly be different; we have seen a handful of such patients who fare a bit better on pimozide than on their earlier antipsychotics. Other than the cardiac effects, the side-effect profile is probably much like haloperidol. Pimozide should cause tardive dyskinesia, but we know of no reported cases. If doses over the FDA's upper limit of 10 mg a day are to be used, an ECG should be obtained after every dosage increase. The drug should probably not be given together with tricyclics, which also alter cardiac function.

In this era of minimal-dose neuroleptic treatment, a trial of pimozide up to 10 mg a day could be carried out in rehospitalized schizophrenic patients. The drug is widely used in some European countries. The dosage equivalency to chlorpromazine is probably 3 mg of pimozide to 100 mg of chlorpromazine.

Haloperidol Decanoate

Depot haloperidol is now readily available as an alternative to depot fluphenazine. It is claimed that its half-life is long enough so that injections every 4 weeks are adequate. Fluphenazine decanoate is often given every 2–3 weeks, but there is no study showing that depot haloperidol every 4 weeks is more effective than depot fluphenazine every 4 weeks, a not uncommon time interval for the latter drug.

If one assumes that 60–70% of orally ingested haloperidol actually survives passage through the gut and the liver to become bioavailable, then a monthly injection of 20 times the daily oral dose is indicated. If a patient is treated with 10 mg of haloperidol a day, 200 mg of haloperidol decanoate a month could be given. The comparable conversion figure for fluphenazine is much lower—12.5 mg (0.5 ml) of the decanoate form every 3 weeks for patients on 10 mg of oral fluphenazine a day. Our guess is that a lower haloperidol decanoate conversion figure will eventually prove adequate.

In the few controlled studies comparing the two depot drugs, haloperidol has tended to be slightly more effective with slightly fewer extrapyramidal side effects. Local experience with haloperidol decanoate is too limited to be helpful. The clinician working in a setting where depot neuroleptics are commonly used should probably try depot haloperidol in a few patients and make up his or her own mind about its utility and consumer acceptance. If haloperidol blood levels prove clinically useful and if blood level data from oral haloperidol studies generalize to patients on depot haloperidol—two big ifs—then depot haloperidol would have an advantage over depot fluphenazine.

In the interim, the extensive research on the maintenance dosages of fluphenazine decanoate required to keep schizophrenic patients reasonably stable in the community makes this older depot drug a better understood treatment modality.

Clozapine

As of this writing, clozapine has just been released by the FDA for use in patients with treatment-resistant schizophrenia or patients who are unable to tolerate the side effects of standard neuroleptics. Clozapine is in many ways the best new development in the treatment of schizophrenia since chlorpromazine was discovered. The drug has problems and dangers. It does not work for everyone, and patients who are helped substantially may still be far from well. However, it is the only antipsychotic drug so far that in controlled studies has been shown to be clearly more effective than older standard neuroleptics and the only antipsychotic so far that causes essentially no pseudoparkinsonism or dystonia and at least much less akathisia. It appears unlikely to cause tardive dyskinesia.

Clozapine has been in clinical use in Europe for over 15 years. It was withdrawn from general use after deaths from agranulocytosis were reported in Finland in the mid-1970s. Over the intervening years, no other antipsychotic with similar properties has been found, perhaps because clozapine has an odd mix of pharmacological effects: more dopamine-1 than dopamine-2 effects; more effect on cortical and limbic dopamine systems than on the basal ganglia; and greater serotonergic ($5-HT_2$), histaminic (H), and alpha-adrenergic blocking activity than other available neuroleptics.

Evidence from old (pre-1978) multicenter trials showed clozapine to be more effective than haloperidol or chlorpromazine, leading Sandoz Pharmaceuticals to remarket the drug under controlled conditions in some European countries. In the United States, the FDA insisted that clozapine's efficacy in demonstrably treatment-resistant schizophrenic patients be proved. This was done, and the resulting study has been published. Chronic schizophrenic patients who had failed on at least three adequate neuroleptic trials and had not had a remission in 5 years were studied. About one-third improved after 4 weeks on clozapine, compared to 2% on chlorpromazine (Kane et al. 1988).

Because of its tendency to cause serious agranulocytosis—affecting about 1.6% of all treated patients in the United States—clozapine is being marketed under a unique system whereby a national home health care agency is the only source of the drug and will be responsible for obtaining weekly white blood cell counts on all patients, essentially forever. Weekly supplies of clozapine are delivered at the time the blood is drawn. This makes the treatment relatively expensive (about $9,000/year). However, because the onset of agranulocytosis is unpredictable—some patients show slow, steady decreases in white blood cell levels, whereas others abruptly plunge into agranulocytosis—the purpose is to catch all new cases rapidly and to institute medical treatment early to avoid the deaths observed in Europe before this adverse effect had been recognized. No deaths have occurred in the United States under weekly monitoring, although some of the patients have become quite febrile and seriously ill. The agranulocytosis is believed to be an autoimmune reaction, not a direct toxic effect on the bone marrow. It is not dose related, and most cases occur in the 2nd through 4th months of treatment, but some reactions have occurred as late as a year and a half after the drug was begun. Patients developing agranulocytosis once will develop it rapidly again if the drug is restarted.

Clozapine is available in both 25-mg and 100-mg scored tablets. The starting dose is 25 mg at bedtime, with twice-a-day dosing recommended by the manufacturer, but many patients will end up taking the whole dose at bedtime. The dose should be increased slowly and cautiously from 25 mg/day to 200 mg/day over the first 2 weeks, then stabilized there for a week with further increases as tolerated. Many patients respond well to daily doses between 200 and 500 mg/day. If clear improvement has not occurred, the dose can be gradually increased to 900 mg/day. However, because drug-related grand mal seizures occur quite frequently (in about 15% of patients) at dosages over 550 mg/day, anticonvulsants should probably be added. Dilantin, in standard anticonvulsant doses, has been used for this purpose at McLean Hospital.

Sedation is one major side effect limiting dosage escalation. Many patients develop tolerance to this effect, but some do not. Cardiovascular side effects, both severe orthostatic hypotension and marked tachycardia up to 130–140 beats/minute, can occur early in clozapine treatment. These side effects require very slow dosage increases and, sometimes, the use of counteractive medications. A few patients develop unpleasant gastrointestinal distress and flulike symptoms early in treatment and refuse to take the drug again. Drug-induced fevers in the 100°F range can occur early in treatment. These pass and are not serious. Blood counts should be obtained, but in local experience with over 75 patients, they have always been normal or elevated. Hypersalivation at night causing wet pillowcases is common. Enuresis occasionally occurs.

Although the manufacturer has strongly urged that patients be taken off other neuroleptics before clozapine is begun, this advice is hard to follow in many psychotic patients. We have often added low doses of clozapine to ongoing antipsychotic therapy, then tapered the prior antipsychotic once the clozapine dose was up to 200 mg/day.

We have combined clozapine generally without incident with benzodiazepines, lithium, valproic acid, tricyclic antidepressants, trazodone, and fluoxetine and even electroconvulsive therapy. Our one case of NMS on clozapine occurred in a patient with a prior history of NMS who was also on lithium. As indicated above, lithium is sometimes thought to predispose patients to NMS. Drugs that are known to induce agranulocytosis—like carbamazepine—should be avoided.

The course of improvement with clozapine treatment is a bit unpredictable. Patients who clearly show a substantial decrease in psychotic symptoms may do so in the first few weeks of treatment or as late as 3–6 months. Some patients, a third or more in our experience, are markedly improved though most are not totally free of psychotic residua. Schizoaffective patients may improve more completely than schizophrenic patients, although schizoaffective patients often have better remissions before clozapine treatment. Patients who are on clozapine for 1 or more years may show gradual, continuing improvement.

Even minimally improved patients may be less impulsively angry, violent, or argumentative and may show a gratifying absence of distressing akathisia, parkinsonism, or akinesia. At McLean Hospital, many such patients have been continued on clozapine because they are less distressed by their symptoms and are less of a management problem even though they are still grossly impaired by psychotic symptoms.

Tardive dyskinesia may be unchanged by clozapine treatment but often fades over time to near the vanishing point. In some patients, the dyskinesia improves early, in others only very slowly. It is unclear whether clozapine suppresses dyskinesia or allows it to fade as it might in patients no longer taking neuroleptics.

Long-term side effects of maintenance clozapine therapy are not known, although in the United States, a handful of patients have been on the drug continuously for over 10 years without known adverse effects (including tardive dyskinesia). With long-term treatment with clozapine, some patients gain weight while others lose a little weight. Our impression is that patients who improve a lot are less likely to gain weight.

The major problem in monitoring clozapine therapy over time is the necessity of keeping alert to decreases in the leukocyte count. Our experience suggests that a fair number of patients will worry the clinician by regularly, or occasionally for a few weeks, running white blood cell counts between 3,000 and 4,200. Others will show dramatic decreases, say from 8,000 to 5,000, from one week to the next. In patients who appear to be benefiting from treatment or who have not been on clozapine long enough for the outcome to be at all clear, we have gone to twice-weekly blood counts until the count has risen again. Getting several weekly blood counts before starting clozapine treatment helps the physician identify patients who are likely to run low leukocyte counts even in the absence of clozapine. One worries less about such patients if the low count is a known characteristic. Should clear agranulocytosis occur or should the count drop below 3,000, the drug should be stopped.

In our opinion, clozapine is useful in all patients requiring neuroleptics who have failed to respond to several other antipsychotics, in those with tardive dyskinesia, and in those with severe, uncontrollable extrapyramidal side effects, especially akathisia, on low doses of several standard antipsychotics.

The cost of the monitoring system plus the drug is relatively high, approximately $9,000 a year. Whether the full costs will be covered by Medicaid, Medicare, or commercial health insurance carriers is unclear at this writing, and the fiscal cost-benefit ratio for patients in public institutions has not been systematically determined. Sandoz Pharmaceuticals assumes that the total monitoring package will be considered a drug cost for third-party payment purposes. All this will doubtless become clearer over time. As of this writing, approximately half the states had approved Medicaid payment for clozapine.

Other Antipsychotic Drugs

A number of other neuroleptic agents are available for prescription use in one or more European countries. Some have been available in Europe for years but have never been released in the United States. A few failed to pass our FDA's carcinogenicity screen; we believe this is true of sulpiride and penfluridol. Fluspirilene, a long-acting injectable drug, is held in suspension by a chemical not approved by our FDA. Some European neuroleptics may never be studied in the United States.

One of the more interesting of the drugs is penfluridol, an antipsychotic that is said to be very long acting and that can be given orally once a week. In many ways, such an agent would be particularly useful in private office settings, rather than an injectable neuroleptic given every 2–4 weeks.

Perphenazine enanthate would be handy for use, if only as an alternative to fluphenazine and haloperidol depot forms. Our understanding is that the two companies initially holding patents on the perphenazine and the enanthate/decanoate ends of the molecule could not come to an agreement to produce this formulation.

Pipotiazine palmitate and fluspirilene are two other depot neuroleptics available in Europe. They appear similar to fluphenazine decanoate. Flupentixol decanoate may be the most interesting of the long-acting injectable preparations. Flupentixol is suspected of having clearer antidepressant properties than the other neuroleptics, and at least one double-blind 6-month study in repeatedly suicidal depressive out-patients demonstrated flupentixol to be more effective than placebo. This drug is on the market in Canada in both oral tablet (0.5 mg) and long-acting injectable forms. The oral antidepressant dose is less than 3 mg/day. The antipsychotic dose is over 3 mg/day.

Sulpiride is clearly an "atypical antipsychotic" in that it is different from the older antipsychotics in its pharmacology. However, it causes enough pseudoparkinsonism, akathisia, galactorrhea, and tardive dyskinesia to make its advantages over other neuroleptics more readily available in the United States unclear. There are several drugs available in Europe that are clinically and pharmacologically related to sulpiride. One of these, metaclopramide (Reglan), is marketed in the United States for gastrointestinal diseases but is probably effective in psychosis and certainly can cause typical neuro-logical side effects and tardive dyskinesia. Most sulpiride-like drugs are good antiemetics and speed peristalsis, including stomach emptying, making them useful in dyspepsia.

A very old phenothiazine, levomepromazine, is widely used in Europe. It is a very sedating neuroleptic, is commonly given at bedtime, and may be less likely to cause neurological side effects. It has analgesic effects and is available in the United States only as an injection for pain.

The reason for discussing these drugs in an American psychopharmacology text is that current FDA and customs policy, influenced by pressures from AIDS patients, allows 3-month supplies of drugs not available in the United States to be imported to treat treatment-resistant patients. It is not clear that any of these drugs are so different and so superior (as was clearly the case with clomipramine in obsessive-compulsive disorder) as to impel many psychiatrists to arrange to bring one or more of these drugs to the United States to treat their patients, but in special situations this might be worth doing.

ALTERNATIVES TO NEUROLEPTIC THERAPY

There are currently no reliable, safe, and effective drug therapies for schizophrenic disorders that can replace dopamine-blocking neuroleptics.

Electroconvulsive therapy can reverse psychotic excitements and catatonic stupor but has no real value in preventing future episodes of psychosis. Reserpine has a weak antipsychotic effect that is slow in onset; even at 10–15 mg a day, major improvement may be delayed for 2 months, and schizophrenic patients may pass through a stage of behavioral turbulence before improving. Such a prospect is clinically discouraging, to say the least. The most positive old studies gave 10 mg im of reserpine daily during the first month. Today, high oral doses are cumbersome. Reserpine at 10 mg/day means having the patient swallow forty 0.25-mg tablets. Worse, a few early cases of dyskinesia were induced by reserpine. Lithium can ameliorate schizophrenic symptoms or suppress episodic violence in schizophrenic patients, but it almost never is an adequate drug therapy by itself. Carbamazepine also ameliorates symptoms in some treatment-resistant psychotic patients when added to a neuroleptic, as a double-blind Israeli study shows (Klein et al. 1984), but it is not, by itself, an adequate therapy for schizophrenia.

Recently, diazepam alone has been reported by both Canadian and German groups to rapidly control psychotic symptoms in small numbers of paranoid schizophrenic patients at doses between 70 and 400 mg a day (the German group used 50-mg tablets). Sedation was *not* a problem, allegedly, after the first day, and improvement continued for 4 weeks. Neither study reported follow-up data. In one study, high-dose diazepam aggravated schizoaffective symptoms. These small, brief studies are intriguing but do not offer a real and useful pharmacological alternative to the standard antipsychotics.

There have now been at least seven reports on the use of alprazolam in neuroleptic-treated schizophrenic patients. Two of the studies involve patients with clear panic attacks as well as chronic psychosis. Both small studies find alprazolam useful in suppressing episodes of panic. Several other small studies, mainly in inpatients, find the addition of alprazolam beneficial in some patients. The original hypothesis was that alprazolam would be particularly useful in treating negative symptoms, but the studies show effects of alprazolam on both positive and negative symptoms in some patients. The only large placebo-controlled study in schizophrenic outpatients was completely negative (Csernansky et al. 1988); neither diazepam nor alprazolam was more effective than placebo over the course of this 8-week trial.

It may be too early to really understand this area, but a reasonable presumption is that alprazolam might help as an adjunct to neuroleptic treatment in patients with panic attacks or other significant anxiety symptoms.

Propranolol has been studied for many years in the treatment of acute and chronic schizophrenia in very high dosages (600–2,000 mg a day) given alone or with a neuroleptic drug. Although Yorkston et al. have reported efficacy in controlled studies, other investigators have found equivocal results with only occasional patients showing any benefit. Since two deaths have occurred on this treatment, one of a silent bleeding peptic ulcer and one sudden death of unknown etiology, this use cannot be generally recommended. However, more recent clinical studies of doses up to 400 mg a day in organically impaired psychiatric patients with impulsive violence or aggression suggest that propranolol may be useful in such patients in controlling temper outbursts, although it does not affect the other underlying behavioral organic deficits.

If such therapy were to be attempted, the relevant articles should be reviewed and dosage increased slowly, with blood pressure and pulse monitoring before each dose until the patient is well stabilized at a constant, effective dose. Propranolol has been reported to increase chlorpromazine blood levels and may do so for other antipsychotics as well.

It is possible that carbamazepine and lithium also offer more promise in the treatment of disturbed behavior in brain damaged, demented, or mentally retarded patients than do the standard antipsychotics, but it is too early to make specific claims or recommendations in these areas. It *is* possible to assert that clinicians who use standard antipsychotics in such nonschizophrenic patients are at risk for criticism or possibly for a malpractice suit if they cannot convincingly document the rationale on which the drug use is based and if they cannot document that the antipsychotic was, in fact, clinically useful in the particular patient treated.

Bibliography

Ayd F: Lorazepam update: 1977–1985. International Drug Therapy Newsletter 20:33–36, 1985

Baldessarini RJ, Cole JO, Davis JM, et al: Tardive Dyskinesia [Task Force Report No 18]. Washington, DC, American Psychiatric Association, 1980

Baldessarini R, Cohen B, Teicher M: Pharmacological treatment, in Schizophrenia: Treatment of Acute Psychotic Episodes. Edited by Levy S, Ninan P. American Psychiatric Press, Washington, DC, 1990, pp 61–118

Beckmann H, Haas S: High dose diazepam in schizophrenia. Psychopharmacology 71:79–82, 1980

Bishop M, Simpson G, Dunnett C, et al: Efficacy of loxapine in the treatment of paranoid schizophrenia. Psychopharmacology 51:107–114, 1977

Blackwell B: Patient compliance with drug therapy. N Engl J Med 289:249–252, 1973

Brown W, Laughren T: Low serum prolactin and early relapse following neuroleptic withdrawal. Am J Psychiatry 138:237–239, 1981

Carpenter W, Heinrichs D: Early intervention, time-limited targeted pharmacotherapy of schizophrenia. Schizophr Bull 9:533–542, 1983

Cohen BM: The clinical utility of plasma neuroleptic levels, in Guidelines for the Use of Psychotropic Drugs. Edited by Stancer H. New York, Spectrum Publications, 1984, pp 245–260

Cole JO: Antipsychotic drugs: is more better? McLean Hospital Journal 7:61–87, 1982

Cole JO, Gardos G: Alternatives to neuroleptic drug therapy. McLean Hospital Journal 10:112–127, 1985

Cole JO, Gardos G, Gelernter J, et al: Supersensitivity psychosis. McLean Hospital Journal 9:46–72, 1984

Comaty JE, Janicak PG: Depot neuroleptics. Psychiatric Annals 17:491–496, 1987

Creese I: Dopamine and antipsychotic medications, in Psychiatry Update: American Psychiatric Association Annual Review, Vol 4. Edited by Hales RE, Frances AJ. Washington, DC, American Psychiatric Press, 1985, pp 17–36

Csernansky JG, Riney SJ, Lombrozo L, et al: Double-blind comparison of alprazolam, diazepam, and placebo for the treatment of negative schizophrenic symptoms. Arch Gen Psychiatry 45:655–659, 1988

Davis JM: Overview: Maintenance therapy in psychiatry, I: schizophrenia. Am J Psychiatry 132:1237–1245, 1975

Davis RJ, Cummings JL: Clinical variants of tardive dyskinesia. Neuropsychiatry, Neuropsychology, and Behavioral Neurology 1:31–38, 1988

Delay J, Deniker P, Harl J: Utilization therapeutique psychiatrique d'une phenothiazine d'action centrale elective (4560 RP). Ann Med Psychol (Paris) 110:112–117, 1952

Delva N, Letemendia F: Lithium treatment in schizophrenic and schizoaffective disorders. Br J Psychiatry 141:387–400, 1982

Dixon L, Weiden P, Frances AJ, et al: Alprazolam intolerance in stable schizophrenic outpatients. Psychopharmacol Bull 25:213–214, 1989

Donaldson SR, Gelenberg AJ, Baldessarini RJ: The pharmacological treatment of schizophrenia: a progress report. Schizophr Bull 9:504–527, 1983

Douyon R, Angrist B, Peselow E, et al: Neuroleptic augmentation with alprazolam: clinical effects and pharmacokinetic correlates. Am J Psychiatry 146:231–234, 1989

Finnerty RJ, Goldberg HL, Nathan L, et al: Haloperidol in neurotic outpatients. Diseases of the Nervous System 37:621–624, 1976

Galbrecht CR, Klett CJ: Predicting response to phenothiazines: the right drug for the right patient. J Nerv Ment Dis 147:173–183, 1968

Gardos G, Casey D: Tardive Dyskinesia and Affective Disorders. Washington, DC, American Psychiatric Press, 1984

Gardos G, Perenyi A, Cole J: Polypharmacy revisited. McLean Hospital Journal 5:178–195, 1980

Garza-Trevino ES, Hollister LE, Overall JE, et al: Efficacy of combinations of intramuscular antipsychotics and sedative-hypnotics for control of psychotic agitation. Am J Psychiatry 146:1598–1601, 1989

Gelenberg H, Mandel M: Catatonic reactions to high potency neuroleptic drugs. Arch Gen Psychiatry 34:947–952, 1977

Greendyke R, Schuster D, Wooten J: Propranolol in the treatment of assaultive patients with organic brain disease. J Clin Psychopharmacol 4:282–285, 1984

Hayes P, Schulz C: The use of beta-adrenergic blocking drugs in anxiety disorders and schizophrenia. Pharmacotherapy 3:101–117, 1983

Herz M, Szymanski H, Simon J: Intermittent medication for stable schizophrenic outpatients. Am J Psychiatry 139:918–922, 1982

Hogarty G: Treatment and course of schizophrenia. Schizophr Bull 3:587–599, 1977

Hogarty GE, Ulrich RJ: Temporal effects of drugs and placebo in delaying relapse in schizophrenic outpatients. Arch Gen Psychiatry 34:297–301, 1977

Jefferson J, Greist J: Haloperidol and lithium: their combined use and the issue of their compatability, in Haloperidol Update, 1958–1980. Edited by Ayd F. Baltimore, MD, Ayd Medical Communications, 1980

Kane J, Woerner M, Weinhold P, et al: A prospective study of tardive dyskinesia: preliminary results. J Clin Psychopharmacol 2:345–349, 1982

Kane JM, Rifkin A, Woerner M, et al: Low dose neuroleptic treatment of outpatient schizophrenics. Arch Gen Psychiatry 40:896, 1983

Kane J, Honigfeld G, Singer J, et al: Clozapine for the treatment-resistant schizophrenic: a double-blind comparison with chlorpromazine. Arch Gen Psychiatry 45:789–796, 1988

Keck PE Jr, Pope HG Jr, Cohen BM, et al: Risk factors for neuroleptic malignant syndrome: a case-control study. Arch Gen Psychiatry (in press)

Keepers GA, Clappison VJ, Casey DE: Initial anticholinergic prophylaxis for neuroleptic-induced extrapyramidal syndromes. Arch Gen Psychiatry 40:113, 1983

Klein E, Bental E, Lerer B, et al: Carbamazepine and haloperidol v placebo and haloperidol in excited psychosis. Arch Gen Psychiatry 41:165–172, 1984

Levenson J: Neuroleptic malignant syndrome. Am J Psychiatry 142:1137–1145, 1985

Lieberman J, Kane J, Johns C: Clozapine guidelines for clinical management. J Clin Psychopharmacol 50:329–338, 1989

Lingjaerde O: Benzodiazepines in the treatment of schizophrenia, in The Benzodiazepines: From Molecular Biology to Clinical Practice. Edited by Costa E. New York, Raven, 1983, pp 369–381

Lipinski JF, Zubenko G, Cohen BM, et al: Propranolol in the treatment of neuroleptic-induced akathisia. Am J Psychiatry 141:412–415, 1984

Luby E: Reserpine-like drugs—clinical efficacy, in Psychopharmacology: A Review of Progress, 1957–1967. Edited by Efron D. Washington, DC, U.S. Government Printing Office, 1968, pp 1077–1082

Marder SR, Van Putten T: Who should receive clozapine? Arch Gen Psychiatry 45:865–867, 1988

Marder SR, Hubbard JW, Van Putten T, et al: Pharmacokinetics of long-acting injectable neuroleptic drugs: clinical implications. Psychopharmacology 98:433–439, 1989

Mason AS, Granacher RP: Clinical Handbook of Antipsychotic Drug Therapy. New York, Brunner/Mazel, 1978

May PRA: Treatment of Schizophrenia: A Comparative Study of Five Treatment Methods. New York, Science House, 1968

Owen RR, Cole JO: Molindone hydrochloride: a review of laboratory and clinical findings. J Clin Psychopharmacol 9:268–276, 1989

Owen RR, Beake BJ, Marby D, et al: Response to clozapine in chronic psychotic patients. Psychopharmacol Bull 25:253–256, 1989

Pisciotta AV: Agranulocytosis induced by certain phenothiazine derivatives. JAMA 208:1862–1868, 1969

Robertson M, Trimble M: Major tranquilizers used as antidepressants—a review. J Affective Disord 4:173–193, 1982

Roy-Byrne P, Gerner R, Liston E, et al: ECT for acute mania: a forgotten treatment modality. Journal of Psychiatric Treatment and Evaluation 3:83–86, 1981

Salam S, Kilzieh N: Lorazepam treatment of psychogenic catatonia. J Clin Psychiatry 49 (suppl):16–21, 1988

Salzman C: The use of ECT in the treatment of schizophrenia. Am J Psychiatry 137:1032–1041, 1980

Silver J, Yudofsky S: Propranolol for aggression: literature review and clinical guidelines. International Drug Therapy Newsletter 20:9–12, 1985

Siris SG, Morgan V, Fagerstrom R, et al: Adjunctive imipramine in the treatment of postpsychotic depression: a controlled trial. Arch Gen Psychiatry 42:533–539, 1987

Teicher MH, Glod CA, Aaronson ST, et al: Open assessment of the safety and efficacy of thioridazine in the treatment of patients with borderline personality disorder. Psychopharmacol Bull 25:535–549, 1989

Tuason V, Escobar J, Garvey M, et al: Loxapine vs chlorpromazine in paranoid schizophrenia. J Clin Psychiatry 45:158–163, 1984

Van Putten T: Why do schizophrenic patients refuse to take their drugs? Arch Gen Psychiatry 31:67–72, 1978

Wojcik J: Antiparkinson drug use. Biological Therapies in Psychiatry Newsletter 2:5–7, 1979

Wolkowitz OM, Breier A, Doran A, et al: Alprazolam augmentation of the antipsychotic effects of fluphenazine in schizophrenic patients: preliminary results. Arch Gen Psychiatry 45:664–671, 1988

Yorkston N, Zaki S, Havard C: Some practical aspects of using propranolol in the treatment of schizophrenia, in Propranolol and Schizophrenia. Edited by Roberts E, Amacher P. New York, Alan R Liss, 1978, pp 83–97

Mood Stabilizers

5

The term "mood stabilizer" was first applied to the lithium salts when it became clear that these compounds not only were effective in manic excitement but also tended to avert both manic and depressive recurrences in bipolar patients. More recently, several anticonvulsants—carbamazepine, valproic acid, and probably clonazepam—have been shown to be effective in the treatment of manic excitement and may have longer-term mood-stabilizing effects in some bipolar or schizoaffective patients. This chapter will consider the properties of lithium salts first and then the use of anticonvulsants in bipolar and related disorders.

LITHIUM

History and Indications

Lithium, usually as the carbonate and occasionally as the citrate salt, is widely used in American psychiatry, particularly considering that its only FDA-approved indications are for the treatment of mania and as maintenance therapy to prevent or diminish the intensity of "subsequent episodes in those manic-depressive patients with a history of mania." As will be discussed below, lithium is often used in patients with a variety of recurrent episodic illnesses with or without prominent affective features. It is also used in patients with mood lability, with impulsive or episodic violence or anger, or even with paramenstrual dysphoria, alcoholism, borderline personality disorder, chronic schizophrenia, and almost any other condition that does not respond to other drug therapies.

The use of lithium salts in psychiatry was initiated by John Cade (an Australian state hospital superintendent) in the 1940s for ultimately irrelevant reasons, but it proved to be an effective though toxic treatment. The addition of serum level monitoring made the treatment safe and provided the first general use of blood level monitoring for a psychiatric drug. The use of lithium in psychiatry generally increased worldwide, although the United States was slow to participate because of an earlier disastrous experience in this country with the unmonitored use of lithium chloride as a salt substitute, which had led to severe toxic reactions, some fatal.

Schou was the first to report compelling evidence that the use of lithium carbonate reduced the incidence and duration of serious affective episodes dramatically in bipolar patients. Since that time, a large number of controlled, double-blind studies have confirmed that lithium is clearly effective in reducing recurrences in both bipolar and unipolar affective disorders, as well as being more effective than placebo in acute mania.

Preparations

Lithium is available in the United States in several formulations (Table 5-1). The standard and least expensive form is the carbonate in 300-mg capsules or scored tablets. Sustained-release preparations of the carbonate are also available as is

Table 5-1. Mood stabilizers

Generic name	Brand name	Formulations
lithium carbonate*†	Eskalith	Tablet: 300 mg
		Capsule: 300 mg
	Lithane	Tablet: 300 mg
	Lithotabs	Tablet: 300 mg
	Eskalith CR (sustained release)	Tablet: 450 mg
	Lithobid (sustained release)	Tablet: 300 mg
lithium citrate	Cibalith-S	8 meq/5 ml (480-ml bottle)
carbamazepine*	Tegretol	Tablet: 200 mg
		Chewable tablet: 100 mg
		Suspension: 100 mg/5 ml (450-ml bottle)
valproic acid*	Depakene	Capsule: 250 mg
		Syrup: 250 mg/5 ml (16-oz bottle)
	Depakote	Enteric-coated tablet: 125, 250, 500 mg
clonazepam	Klonopin	Tablet: 0.5, 1.0, 2.0 mg

*Available in generic form.
†A generic preparation by Roxane is available in 300-mg scored tablets and 150-, 300-, and 600-mg capsules.

a liquid preparation of lithium citrate; in the latter case, one teaspoonful is the equivalent of the ion content of 300 mg of the carbonate (8 meq). Other preparations, including the sulfate, and other dosage strengths are used in Europe. Despite over 30 years of clinical experience with lithium, it is not entirely clear whether any of the formulations have clear superiority for any purpose except that the citrate is obviously useful in patients who dislike or cannot swallow pills.

The sustained-release preparations result in lower peak serum lithium levels after ingestion and probably result in less lithium ion being released in the stomach and more in the small intestine. If lithium irritation of the stomach mucosa is causing nausea after each dose, then the sustained-release preparation might reduce gastric irritation. If diarrhea is a problem (and is not due to an elevated serum lithium level), then the citrate might cause even faster absorption in the upper gastrointestinal tract and might reduce the diarrhea. However, we have seen patients with diarrhea on standard lithium carbonate whose diarrhea lessened on sustained-release lithium.

The basic problem is that it is still unclear which lithium side effects are related to peak serum level and which to steady-state serum level. Clinically, any side effect that mainly occurs 1–2 hours after each oral dose of the standard preparation might be improved by the sustained-release form. For example, nausea may be caused by lithium's gastric irritation or by an elevated serum level. The former would cause transient nausea after each dose; the latter would cause persistent nausea.

There was a belief that sustained-release lithium would, in general, cause fewer side effects and might cause, in particular, less effect on the concentrating ability of the renal tubules, leading to less polyuria and polydipsia. So far, this does not seem to be the case, and it may even be that massing the total lithium daily dose at bedtime may cause fewer renal effects. One major European center (Copenhagen) routinely has been using once-a-day lithium dosage for many years, suggesting that this dosage scheme is feasible and effective.

As noted below, sometimes lithium causes skin rashes that appear to be allergic in nature; these may be due to other ingredients in a particular lithium preparation and may disappear if a different preparation is substituted.

Blood Levels

Lithium dosage is titrated to achieve both therapeutic response and "adequate" blood levels. The general presumption is that levels of around 0.7–1.0 meq/L are appropriate for maintenance therapy or the treatment of conditions other than manic or psychotic excitement, whereas levels up to 1.5 meq/L are sometimes needed in acute mania. Levels should be obtained about 12 hours after the last dose, at which time the vagaries of absorption after drug ingestion are well past and a relative steady state has been achieved (see the section "Tricyclic Blood Levels" in Chapter 3). These "ideal" levels are, of course, not carved in stone and must be interpreted in the clinical context. Someone who has marked tremor, oversedation, vomiting, and ataxia at a level of 0.8 meq/L either cannot tolerate that level or has some other medical condition causing the symptoms, with lithium intolerance being more likely. Other patients on maintenance therapy appear to have averted affective episodes for years at levels as low as 0.4–0.6 meq/L, and patients with daily symptoms such as irritability and anger claim clinical improvement at very low blood levels. It is very hard to prove that these are (or are not) "real" drug responses. It is our belief that many patients can be successfully maintained at relatively low serum levels. Occasionally, a patient whose mania is still uncontrolled despite a level of 1.5 meq/L for several days and has no side effects could be cautiously tried at a higher level.

Clinical Use Patterns

Lithium use can be divided into four general clinical contexts:

1. To control rapidly acute, overt psychopathology as in mania or psychotic agitation
2. To attempt to modify milder ongoing or frequent but episodic clinical symptoms such as chronic depression or episodic irritability
3. To establish a prophylactic maintenance regimen to avert future affective or psychotic episodes
4. To enhance the effect of antidepressants in patients with major depressive episodes (see Chapters 3 and 9)

Acute psychosis. Rapid establishment of high, adequate lithium levels (e.g., 0.8–1.2 meq/L) is desired for acute psychosis, and an initial regimen of 300 mg two to four times a day is indicated in healthy adolescent or adult patients with lithium serum levels obtained every 3 or 4 days initially, to ensure early detection of toxic lithium levels. The dose is titrated up (or down) as necessary to achieve a level of approximately 1.0 meq/L. In patients over 60 or those with possible renal impairment, the lower starting dose is indicated. Response in acutely manic states may require 5–14 days to occur, even with adequate blood levels. As blood levels stabilize, their frequency may be decreased to two times a week initially and eventually to once a week as both blood levels and the clinical condition level out. If no clinical response occurs within 4 weeks, it is safe to assume that lithium will not be effective in the acute episode.

In practice, because lithium alone is not enough in excited manic patients, most acutely psychotic patients will be on antipsychotic drugs concurrently, prior to lithium therapy, or will have antipsychotics added if lithium does not have some obvious clinical effect in the first week. This combined therapy will, of course, confound the clinician's ability to judge whether lithium is having a significant clinical effect.

Other Current Target Symptoms

For other target symptoms, the situation is less urgent and an initial dosage of 300 mg twice a day seems adequate. There are some patients who end up benefiting from lithium who present with histories of marked lithium intolerance that appears to have been caused by overaggressive initial dosing. In these less urgent situations, a blood level of 0.5–0.8 meq/L is probably adequate, and less frequent blood levels are needed. It is also important to remember that one is treating a patient, not a blood level, and that both clinical status and side effects need frequent careful monitoring. Some patients report clear symptom relief at levels around 0.5 meq/L; it seems senseless to push them to higher serum levels.

Similarly, keeping a patient chronically nauseated, mentally dulled, and grossly tremulous just to maintain an "adequate" blood level is counterproductive in almost all situations.

In chronic disorders manifesting overt current target psychopathology—depression, schizophrenia, cyclothymic frequent mood shifts, irascibility with frequent temper outbursts—trials of about 4 weeks with adequate or highest tolerated blood levels are usually sufficient to determine whether lithium will be clinically useful.

Maintenance Therapy

In patients who are in remission and are being stabilized on lithium to avert future psychotic episodes, one can begin at even lower dosages (one or two 300-mg doses a day); weekly serum levels are often sufficient during dosage adjustment. Again, the goal is to find a well-tolerated blood level as close to 0.8 meq/L as possible. It is still unclear whether better prophylaxis occurs at higher serum levels. It seems reasonable that it should, and, in one major National Institute of Mental Health (NIMH) collaborative study, patients maintained at 0.8 meq/L and above had fewer recurrences than patients stabilized at lower levels.

However, many clinicians report satisfactory prophylaxis at lower levels in some patients. Once a patient on maintenance lithium is stabilized adequately with weekly serum levels for a few weeks, monthly levels are sufficient, and after 6 months to a year of stability, levels every 3 months may suffice.

Once a patient has a stable daily dose, this can be spread over the day in any suitable regimen. Usually twice a day— morning and bedtime—is convenient and well tolerated, and dosages are less likely to be forgotten or overlooked. It has been suggested, but not proven, that once-a-day dosage may be associated with less polyuria. Gastric irritation after each dose is the major reason for spreading medication into three or four smaller administrations a day. Smaller, more frequent dosages are common (and logistically easy) in hospitalized patients but they are sometimes inadvertently discharged on these regimens when a simpler regimen would suffice and might be taken more reliably after the patient is discharged to home.

Reinstitution of Lithium Therapy

In patients who have responded in the past to lithium but have stopped the drug for weeks or months, it is clinically reasonable to place them immediately back on their prior dosage without retitrating if there is no reason to believe kidney function has changed in the interim. Frequent blood level monitoring should be reinstituted.

Dose Prediction and Dose Requirements

Several articles have described techniques for predicting the optimal dosage of lithium from a loading dose followed by several level determinations over the next 24 hours. These techniques can be used but do not seem to us to be worth the effort.

Specific Clinical Indications

Mania. There is no final, conclusive statement possible about the use of lithium as a sole or primary drug treatment of acute mania. Lithium alone is clearly more effective than placebo and probably as effective as an antipsychotic in less severely excited manic patients. It is probably less effective than an antipsychotic in very hyperactive, disturbed, psychotic manic, or schizoaffective patients. However, given the risk of tardive dyskinesia with antipsychotics, a few clinicians opt to use lithium alone or with other less conventional antimanic agents such as clonazepam, valproic acid, or carbamazepine to avoid antipsychotics. Others start all manic patients routinely on an antipsychotic on the assumption that this will produce the most rapid control of psychopathology or aid in patient management. Many clinicians will then add lithium, either on the first day of drug therapy or after the mania has begun to respond to antipsychotics, to stabilize the patient on both drugs. When the patient is clearly much improved, some clinicians will gradually taper the antipsychotic so that the patient will be on lithium alone at the end of the episode. In patients whose hospitalizations are brief, both medications will be in use at discharge and the antipsychotic will be tapered in the community.

In patients with several prior manic episodes, the past history of drug response may be a guide to treatment of the new episode. On the other hand, in a patient with only a single typical manic episode, one can justify using only an antipsychotic and later instituting lithium if further affective episodes occur.

The problem of severe neurotoxicity, reported mainly with the combined use of haloperidol and lithium in psychotic excitement, deserves comment here. It is usually characterized by gross tremor, confusion, delirium, and sometimes dyskinesia. It can occur with lithium in combination with other neuroleptics. Similar states can occur with lithium toxicity alone. However, this severe complication is very rare and is mainly a reason to observe patients in combination treatment carefully and to stop both drugs at once if severe neurotoxic signs begin to emerge. One suspects that haloperidol-lithium toxicity is relatively more common because haloperidol is widely used in the treatment of mania. Again there is no compelling evidence that haloperidol is more effective than other neuroleptics in mania, and the severe neurotoxicity has been observed on other antipsychotics combined with lithium. If clinicians are seriously concerned about the lithium-haloperidol toxicity, this combination can readily be avoided, but clinical experience suggests that the combination is worth trying if the clinician prefers haloperidol in mania.

Schizophrenia. There is reasonable evidence that lithium, at serum levels in the 0.8–1.1 meq/L range, is useful in combination with an antipsychotic in schizoaffective patients, some of whom are considered atypical bipolar patients. This poorly defined group of conditions includes patients with chronic symptoms of psychosis between episodes as well as patients with reasonably good interepisode adjustment who show florid non-affect-consonant delusions and hallucinations during excited episodes. In both cases, if overactivity, insomnia, pressured speech, irritability, or other common manic symptoms are present during the episode, lithium is a reasonable drug therapy to add to an antipsychotic. In the few controlled studies in which lithium is added to an antipsychotic in schizophrenic patients with or without manic symptoms, lithium is often more effective, on the average, than placebo.

In some chronically impaired schizophrenic patients with no more than the usual amount of affective overlay, lithium will produce useful but limited additional improvement when added to an antipsychotic regimen. This happens often enough to make a trial of lithium easily justifiable in any treatment-resistant schizophrenic patient, although perhaps only one in five will show clinical improvement. There is also a subgroup of chronic schizophrenic patients with brief episodic angry outbursts in whom lithium appears to act by decreasing impulsive anger rather than by reducing the level of psychosis.

However, in chronic treatment-resistant psychotic patients, drug treatments are often added and continued for months or years even if no obvious clinical response or only a trivial improvement has occurred, in the hope that the extra drugs might be helping. There seems little justification for continuing such a use of lithium for longer than 6 months if no clinical benefit is apparent.

Recurrent bipolar disorder. There is excellent evidence that lithium carbonate is more effective than placebo in preventing the recurrence of affective episodes, either manic or depressive, in bipolar patients. However, only half or maybe fewer of such patients have complete suppression of all episodes even with excellent medication compliance. Further, at least some of the patients who have manic recurrences on maintenance lithium are blamed for noncompliance unjustifiably— the noncompliance is probably secondary to a recurrence of mania rather than vice versa. In addition, some patients respond to lithium with suppression of mania but with continuing episodes of depression; others show only a partial reduction in severity in both phases. We have seen several patients who had been on lithium for several years and did badly, continuing to have episodes of mania and depression; they were judged to be lithium nonresponders but were clearly even worse when lithium therapy was abandoned as ineffective. Rapid-cycling bipolar patients generally do less well on lithium than patients with less frequent or regular episodes, but even some of these patients can have the severity of their episodes modulated.

In initiating maintenance "prophylactic" lithium therapy, both patient and, where available, spouse or significant other need careful instruction about the purposes and requirements of lithium therapy and possible side effects and complications. There is evidence that continuing involvement of bipolar patients and their spouses in couples groups or of single patients in lithium support groups is helpful in maintaining intelligent drug compliance and in helping patients handle past, current, and future problems.

Many bipolar patients, when contemplating maintenance lithium therapy, ask, "Will I have to take lithium forever?" There are two issues here. One is whether patients ever stop having recurrent manic and depressive episodes once several episodes have occurred, and the other is whether abruptly stopping lithium will trigger an affective episode that might not otherwise occur. The evidence from placebo substitution studies in patients already stabilized successfully on lithium maintenance is that relapses occur with considerable frequency with about half the patients relapsing within 6 months. Other, uncontrolled studies have reported small series of patients who relapse floridly within a few days. We suspect the latter consequence is unusual but may be real in some patients and may account for some of the florid relapses seen in patients on maintenance lithium who experiment with stopping (or forget to take) their medication for a few days. In our experience, stopping lithium abruptly for 2 or 3 days in patients who have developed uncomfortable symptoms of lithium toxicity has never led to a florid relapse.

The whole area of lithium discontinuation is not well understood, but most clinicians assume that essentially all bipolar patients who are stable on lithium need to continue the medication indefinitely. One wonders, however, whether a trial off lithium could be worth trying in patients who have really stabilized both their illnesses and their life circumstances for several years and in whom there is some evidence that prior episodes were precipitated by stresses that are no longer present. Such trials off lithium need to be discussed in detail with patients and their families. Given the occasional rapid relapses observed on sudden discontinuation, slowly tapering the drug by 300 mg a day each month may be indicated on grounds of general conservativism.

Depressive disorders.   Some depressions improve on lithium alone (and some on placebo alone). Lithium alone has not been proven to be consistently effective in the treatment of depression, but some experts assert that lithium is particularly effective in depressions in bipolar patients. So few bipolar patients are seen these days in a depression and off lithium that this proposition is almost untestable. There are also recent studies suggesting that adding lithium to a tricyclic antidepressant or a monoamine oxidase inhibitor in a patient who has not responded to the antidepressant after 3–6 weeks may lead to a clear, favorable response (see Chapters 3 and 9).

There is some suggestion that mixed affective states with dysphoria, agitation, insomnia, and pressured thoughts and speech may be helped by lithium. It is also worth trying in patients with rapid, unstable mood shifts occurring within a day (emotionally unstable character disorder) or in patients meeting DSM-III-R criteria for cyclothymic disorder.

In patients with bipolar disorder, the evidence is that combining imipramine with lithium in maintenance therapy may slightly increase the risk of manic relapse. In recurrent unipolar depression, the evidence from large-scale studies is mixed on the exact prophylactic potential of lithium; some showed lithium and imipramine to be equally effective, whereas the most recent study showed imipramine to be superior to lithium but both to be superior to placebo. The combination of imipramine and lithium was not superior to imipramine alone. Thus, clinicians may choose to use lithium alone to prevent recurrence of depression.

As a drug useful in episodic affective disorder, lithium has been tried in paramenstrual dysphoria with some success, but the vagueness of the condition and its alleged placebo responsivity make this potential indication a bit suspect.

Rage and irritability. There is a reasonable clinical literature, mainly but not exclusively uncontrolled, that supports the proposition that some patients with episodic, uncontrolled, violent rage outbursts respond to lithium. The drug is certainly not always effective in such cases, but these predominantly nonpsychotic behavior disorders often present such appalling clinical problems that any drug with a chance of helping substantially deserves a trial. We concur with Tupin's general position that in violent prisoners and the like, lithium controls outbursts of rage that are untriggered or triggered instantaneously by minor stimuli; however, lithium does not affect premeditated aggressive behavior. The drug is helpful in some patients with organic disorders or mental retardation who display episodic angry outbursts. It should be noted that there have been a few case reports of lithium causing increased aggressive behavior in patients with temporal lobe spike activity on EEG.

Alcoholism.   There are clinical claims that lithium is useful in episodic, binge drinkers in preventing their dipsomanic episodes. Certainly some patients presenting as alcoholics have underlying bipolar or unipolar recurrent affective disorders and drink to excess to anesthetize their depression or to slow their mania; such patients should benefit from lithium. Early controlled studies by Merry et al. (1976) and by Kline et al. (1974), although weak in their findings, suggested that some alcoholic patients with depressive symptoms do better on lithium than on placebo over time. However, most alcoholic patients show some dysphoria during detoxification, and many have the recall of their past psychiatric histories well muddled by alcoholism; these complications make clear differentiation of affective disorder difficult in chronic alcoholic patients. There are two recent reports that are on the surface contradictory. Fawcett et al. (1987) reported that lithium was effective in preventing relapse of alcoholism. However, Dorns et al. (1989) reported that lithium did not affect the course of alcoholism in either depressed or nondepressed alcoholic patients.

On balance, it seems preferable to reserve lithium therapy for alcoholic patients with a documented history of recurrent bipolar disorder.

Side Effects

Neuromuscular and central nervous system effects.   The most common side effect in lithium therapy is tremor, principally noticed in the fingers. It resembles intention, coffee-induced, or familial tremor in frequency, being faster than pseudoparkinsonian tremor. When tremor is severe enough to affect handwriting, the writing is usually jagged and irregular, but not micrographic as in parkinsonism. Tremor is sometimes worse at peak lithium blood level and can be ameliorated by dosage rearrangement. Dosage reduction can often be used to bring the blood level low enough to make tremor either absent or mild and inconspicuous. If there is good reason to maintain a serum lithium level that causes a disturbing degree of tremor, propranolol at doses from 30 to 160 mg a day can be used to reduce the tremor. Some patients on lithium also develop cogwheeling and mild signs of parkinsonism, and naturally occurring parkinsonism can be aggravated. With toxic lithium levels, gross tremulousness and ataxia with dysarthria will occur, with the patient appearing grossly neurologically disordered and often confused or, less often, delirious at the same time. Seizures occur rarely with severe lithium toxicity.

Some patients on lithium complain of slowed mentation and forgetfulness and, on testing, a memory deficit has been found. Although such patients are often suspected or accused of "using" such symptoms to avoid necessary lithium therapy, our impression is that these complaints are often real and constitute a basis for lowering the dosage or trying another therapy. Some patients worry that they may become less creative on lithium. Schou, however, has asserted that maintenance lithium therapy does not generally affect artistic creativity.

With all of the above neurological symptoms, stopping lithium will lead to a disappearance of the side effects, but the symptoms and signs may persist for 2–5 days, longer than one would think it would take for the offending lithium to be cleared from the body.

Gastrointestinal effects. Chronic nausea and watery diarrhea can occur together or separately as signs of lithium toxicity. Episodic nausea occurring only after each dose may be due to local gastric irritation and may be relieved by taking lithium with food. Shifting to a different lithium preparation may also be helpful. For example, in upper gastrointestinal distress, sustained-release preparations may be beneficial. In contrast, patients with diarrhea who are on sustained-release preparations may benefit from a switch to the shorter-release forms.

Weight gain and endocrine effects. Some patients gain weight progressively on lithium. The mechanisms are unclear. A few patients have overt edema and/or lose several pounds rapidly when lithium is stopped. In more patients, increased appetite with resulting weight gain is the problem, and attempting to control weight with dietary regulation is often very difficult for the patient. Weight gain is greater in patients who are overweight to begin with and is probably greater in patients with polydipsia, perhaps because they drink caloric fluids.

Most patients show a transitory decrease in thyroid levels early in lithium therapy, and a very few show goiter with normal thyroid studies except for elevated thyroid-stimulating hormone levels. Some clinicians add thyroid supplements at this point. However, we recommend using thyroid primarily in patients with marked goiter or in those with associated anergy. Persistent hypothyroidism on lithium can occur but it is rare; it requires thyroid medication.

Renal effects. Lithium causes polyuria with secondary poly-dipsia to a noticeable degree in some patients, roughly perhaps in one out of five. In a few patients this may extend to severe renal diabetes insipidus with urine volume up to 8 liters a day and difficulty in concentrating urine and maintaining adequate lithium serum levels. This range of renal effects is due to a decrease in the resorption of fluid from the distal tubules of the kidney. It can be treated, obviously, by lowering the dose of lithium or stopping the drug. In most, but not all, cases the renal effect wears off in days or weeks after lithium is stopped.

An alternative strategy in patients in whom lithium is clearly necessary and the polyuria is distressing is to add a thiazide diuretic. It is well documented that chlorothiazide at a dose of 500 mg a day decreases lithium clearance by about 50%. Thus one can rationally add 500 mg of chlorothiazide a day and then reduce the lithium dosage by 50% and carefully restabilize the desired lithium level. This maneuver is sometimes effective, as it is in naturally occurring nephrogenic diabetes insipidus, and can be used in milder but troublesome cases of polyuria. At the time of our first edition, amiloride (Midamor) had recently been reported to decrease lithium-induced polyuria without, allegedly, affecting either potassium excretion or lithium serum levels. However, we have seen some patients who show increased lithium levels when amiloride is added. If this is tried, one should check lithium levels carefully while assessing amiloride's effectiveness in improving renal resorption of fluid and decreasing urine volume.

The prohibition in PDR against combining lithium with diuretics, particularly of the thiazide type, is much overstated. If a patient is stabilized on lithium at a clinically useful blood level (e.g., 0.8 meq/L) and a thiazide diuretic is added in ignorance, the lithium level can double and the patient may suddenly develop signs of lithium toxicity. However, we see no problem in starting lithium therapy in a patient already stabilized on a thiazide diuretic; even patients on the artificial kidney have been successfully treated with lithium. Renal impairment before lithium therapy means the clinician should raise the dose very slowly and cautiously with careful serum level monitoring.

A different and potentially more serious renal problem is interstitial nephritis, first reported by Danish workers in

1977. It is characterized by renal scarring and glomerular destruction. Currently, the problem no longer seems as threatening or bothersome as it did initially. Major renal impairment manifested by seriously decreased creatinine clearance appears to be quite rare—we are aware of only a handful of such patients observed at McLean Hospital who had any significant decrease in creatinine clearances since the phenomenon was first described. All but one of these had either serum creatinine levels or creatinine clearances that were only slightly abnormal. Reports from Europe and the United States tend to be confirmatory—no patients with life-threatening kidney dysfunction have been reported. Some patients with chronic affective disorders who have never been on lithium show renal pathology, and not all kidney dysfunction in patients on lithium is necessarily caused by the drug.

Still, it is worth checking kidney function periodically in patients on maintenance lithium. The "best" way would be to measure creatinine clearance periodically, but logistical problems and doubts about patient reliability in 24-hour urine collection have caused this procedure to be generally disfavored. Serum creatinine itself offers a reasonable indicator of kidney function since creatinine production is a function of muscle mass and is not affected by diet. Lithium serum level at constant intake is also a function of glomerular filtration. Watching both measures periodically should allow detection of early changes in glomerular function.

If the lithium dosage requirement gradually decreases and serum creatinine is persistently elevated, then a nephrology consultation is indicated. Even if renal impairment appears to exist, the decision whether to stop lithium therapy should be based on the total situation. Patients who enjoy major benefits from maintenance lithium and have either mild renal deficit or a kidney problem that may not be lithium related can be kept on lithium with more frequent monitoring of kidney function.

Drug effects on lithium excretion. In addition to the effect of thiazide diuretics (or low-salt diets, including fasting completely) in decreasing lithium excretion, xanthine diuretics including caffeine probably *increase* lithium excretion. High coffee intake in hospitalized manic patients could account for the difficulty sometimes encountered in achieving therapeutic serum lithium levels even with very large lithium carbonate dosages (e.g., 2400 mg a day) in such patients.

Indomethacin and phenylbutazone have been reported to significantly decrease lithium excretion in humans; all the newer nonsteroidal anti-inflammatory drugs, including ibuprofen, should be viewed with suspicion. If a patient maintained on lithium requires such drug therapy, lithium levels should be closely monitored and the patient should be observed for possible increases in toxic symptoms. Aspirin clearly does not affect lithium levels and may be the best choice for analgesia or anti-inflammatory action in patients treated with lithium. We could find no information on the effects of acetaminophen. However, we have never had any problems with this combination.

We have seen one patient on lithium who received a course of metronidazole therapy and has, ever since, shown a clear though clinically unimportant increase in serum creatinine into the abnormal range plus a decrease in the dose of lithium needed to maintain her previous serum lithium levels (Teicher et al. 1987). There is another similar case in the literature.

Cardiovascular effects. Cases have been reported in which a "sick sinus node" syndrome has been brought on by lithium. This complication is very rare and probably not predictable unless the condition antedates lithium therapy. Baseline cardiograms are desirable in older patients or patients with any history at all of cardiac dysfunction.

Dermatologic effects. A wide variety of diverse rashes have been described with lithium. Aggravation of preexisting or dormant psoriasis is well documented, and a dry noninflamed papular eruption is relatively common on maintenance lithium. Both zinc sulfate and tetracycline have been tried as treatments for this with variable success. Other less typical (for lithium) rashes of an itchy, presumably allergic nature can occur and often disappear if the specific lithium brand being used is changed; presumably these are allergic reactions to some ingredient in the capsule or tablet other than the lithium itself. Alopecia can occur in patients on lithium, but the hair often regrows either on or off lithium.

Other side effects.   A variety of strange but rare symptoms can occur on lithium that sometimes turn out to be lithium related. At least, they disappear when lithium is stopped and return when it is reinstituted, a reasonable though not infallible test of the drug-relatedness of any odd treatment-emergent symptom or sign on any drug.

Lithium in Pregnancy

Lithium is the only psychoactive nonanticonvulsant drug reliably associated with a specific birth defect, Ebstein's anomaly. This serious cardiac abnormality is not common in children born to mothers on lithium (between 0.1 and 3%), but is much more frequent in lithium babies than in the population at large. Other cardiac defects can also occur in lithium babies, perhaps at a rate as high as 8%. This risk needs to be discussed with female patients on lithium who either are planning to get pregnant or are already pregnant (see Chapter 12). Echocardiography can be used after the 16th week of pregnancy to check for the presence of cardiac abnormalities.

Lithium Information

A lithium information center exists at the University of Wisconsin in Madison. The telephone number is (608) 263–

6171. The staff is most helpful in conducting focused literature searches for a small fee and can provide interested clinicians with helpful answers to a wide variety of questions about lithium problems encountered in their practice.

ANTICONVULSANTS

In the past decade, increasing attention has been paid to the use of classic anticonvulsant medications in psychiatry, mainly to promote mood stabilization. The application of these agents stems from a number of observations on the psychiatric sequelae of temporal lobe epilepsy, including hallucinations, angry outbursts, religiosity, etc. These spurred on the use of phenytoin in the 1950s in psychiatric patients with, at best, equivocal results. In more recent years, several groups have further suggested that psychiatric symptoms could emanate from limbic seizures and that kindling phenomena could play a major role in the development of psychoses and psychiatric disorders. Understandably, then, a number of reports have emerged that other anticonvulsant agents (e.g., carbamazepine and valproic acid), which act more preferentially on temporal lobe or limbic systems, are effective in patients with manic-depressive illness, particularly in acute mania. Three compounds—carbamazepine, valproic acid, and clonazepam—have received the lion's share of attention (for chemical structures, see Figure 5-1), although many of the available anticonvulsants could eventually prove useful in treating mood disorders. Of these, carbamazepine and valproic acid have been best studied as long-term maintenance therapies.

Carbamazepine

Carbamazepine was originally synthesized in 1957 and introduced into the European market in the early 1960s as a treatment for epilepsy, particularly involving the temporal lobes. Subsequently, it became widely used as a treatment

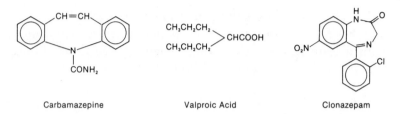

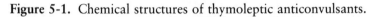

Carbamazepine   Valproic Acid   Clonazepam

Figure 5-1. Chemical structures of thymoleptic anticonvulsants.

for "tic douloureux"—trigeminal neuralgia. Its use for manic-depressive illness stems from the early 1970s when Japanese researchers reported it was effective in many bipolar patients, including patients who were refractory to lithium. In 1980, Ballenger and Post reported that carbamazepine was effective in a double-blind crossover trial in acute bipolar patients. More recently, Kishimoto et al. (1983) reported that it was also effective in maintenance therapy.

Clinical indications.   There are now several controlled studies of carbamazepine in the treatment of acute mania and a few on its maintenance use as a mood stabilizer in bipolar patients. Although neither indication has had the kinds of large American multicenter collaborative trials necessary to convince our FDA of the drug's safety and efficacy for either use, there is enough clinical evidence to justify using carbamazepine in treatment-resistant bipolar patients with a reasonable expectation that a proportion of these, 25–50%, will show clear clinical benefit. The drug does not work any more rapidly than lithium or neuroleptics in acute mania.

Although some responders to carbamazepine improve or stabilize on the drug alone, others do better on carbamazepine plus lithium (see Chapter 9), or carbamazepine plus a neuroleptic. The major problem in assessing the clinical value of a drug like carbamazepine, which is mainly used in seriously symptomatic psychiatric patients who have failed on more standard treatments, is that the patient is rarely taken off all other medications before the carbamazepine is added. Later, if the patient does well, then other preexisting drugs may or may not be tapered and stopped. Clinically, it is often hard to be sure when carbamazepine itself is really working and when prior therapy may finally have begun to work.

There is some evidence that carbamazepine works better than lithium in producing stability in "rapid-cycling" bipolar patients—those with four or more affective episodes a year. There is also evidence that carbamazepine is preferentially effective in more severe paranoid, angry manic patients than in euphoric, overactive, overtalkative, overfriendly manic patients.

Carbamazepine may sometimes be helpful in depression, but it cannot be said to be a potent, reliable first-line therapy. Post and colleagues (1986) have hypothesized that the drug may be more effective than lithium in the treatment of dysphoric mania.

In excited schizophrenic patients there is evidence that, added to the neuroleptic, carbamazepine is of at least short-term benefit. Local experience at McLean Hospital in treatment-resistant schizoaffective and schizophrenic patients suggests that adding carbamazepine to a mélange of other drugs including a neuroleptic is rarely a clear plus. Many such patients are perhaps a little better, but often remain on carbamazepine for months without really showing major improvement. Some patients with an initial positive response lose this effect after a few weeks or months.

A complicating factor in adding carbamazepine to a neuroleptic is that carbamazepine will induce liver enzymes and speed metabolism of some other drugs. Haloperidol levels are clearly lowered substantially. Levels of other antipsychotics could be checked before and 2–4 weeks after carbamazepine is added to see if they are changed. Worsening in some patients (and improvement in others) could be attributed to lowering of the neuroleptic blood level rather than the direct effects of carbamazepine. Similarly, carbamazepine may lower tricyclic antidepressant plasma levels, making such combinations difficult.

Pilot studies of carbamazepine in violent nonpsychotic patients and in alcohol or benzodiazepine withdrawal show some promise in these conditions.

The most intriguing recent study is by Cowdry et al. (1988) and involves patients with borderline personality disorder with histories of frequent impulsive acts. In this small but double-blind study, carbamazepine was notable for substantially decreasing impulsivity. The patients' therapists all judged the patients to be much better. The patients, however, did not feel the drug was doing anything much. In the same study, the patients felt better—but were much more impulsive—on alprazolam.

There is a possibility that carbamazepine might be helpful in nephrogenic diabetes insipidus because it increases vasopressin release. Unfortunately, carbamazepine's ability to do this is blocked by lithium, making carbamazepine ineffective in lithium-induced polyuria and polydipsia. Carbamazepine can, but rarely does, cause hyponatremia and water intoxication.

Is carbamazepine a standard accepted drug therapy for use in psychiatric patients? We believe that the evidence of some efficacy in bipolar patients, both in the manic phase and as a maintenance therapy, is substantial. If one adds to that years of clinical experience with its use with very little evidence of serious adverse effects, then it seems reasonable to endorse carbamazepine as a sensible drug to use in bipolar patients who do not respond to or cannot tolerate lithium. Given this, it is hard to be critical of other less well documented clinical uses of carbamazepine (e.g., for impulsive anger) when other psychiatric drugs (e.g., lithium, tricyclics, antipsychotics) are used well outside their official FDA-approved indications. Nevertheless, the more exotic one's drug use, the more vulnerable one is if serious harm occurs. Documenting why one is using carbamazepine in the chart and documenting verbal or written informed consent from patient or guardian are useful procedures and may help avert malpractice suits should there be adverse consequences.

Dosage schedule. Blood levels of carbamazepine should be monitored at least weekly through the first 8 weeks of treatment because the drug induces liver enzymes, which then speed its own metabolism. The blood level established at 3 weeks may decrease by one-third at 6 weeks, despite the carbamazepine dose being held constant. Starting with 100 mg (one-half tablet) at bedtime is suggested to see if the patient is oversedated. If the drug is well tolerated, 100 mg bid should be given on the second day, followed by 200 mg bid for the next few days. Serum levels should be obtained twice a week in the first 2 weeks where possible, always about 12 hours after the last dose.

Dose should be adjusted to maintain a serum level of 6–8 mg/L. Higher levels are not generally more effective and are often difficult to attain because of hepatic induction. Adjusting levels upward means more risk of side effects. Sedation is the most common problem. Tolerance will often develop. Moving all or most of the daily dose to bedtime may help.

The most common signs of excessive carbamazepine blood levels are diplopia, malcoordination, and sedation.

Side effects. The major concern with the clinical use of carbamazepine is the threat of agranulocytosis or aplastic anemia, potentially lethal conditions. As is usual with very rare, serious adverse drug reactions, estimates of incidence vary widely from 1 case in 10,000 patients treated to a recent estimate of 1 in 125,000 patients. There is much disagreement in the literature as to the need for frequent monitoring of blood counts in patients on carbamazepine. When the drug was a novel treatment in psychiatry, weekly complete blood counts were often recommended, perhaps for the first 6 months, followed by monthly counts thereafter. More recently, British experts have taken the position that regular blood counts are unnecessary and that warning the patient and/or significant others to watch for overt symptoms of bone marrow suppression (e.g., fever, sore throat, petechiae) is more cost-effective (Carbamazepine Update 1989).

Clinical practice with respect to chlorpromazine, where agranulocytosis may be more frequent, has long been to avoid regular blood counts. With clozapine, where the rate of agranulocytosis is perhaps 1–2%, weekly counts have been demanded by the FDA. Obviously, no compelling recommendation is possible with respect to carbamazepine.

One compromise would be to get a complete blood count with every carbamazepine blood level. An ethical and clinical issue here is, "How extra careful should the clinician be using a conceivably dangerous drug outside its approved indications?" This question must be answered separately by each clinical facility and each clinician in private practice. Facilities should have a clear written policy statement that should then be adhered to carefully.

When threatened with malpractice suits, it helps if the clinician (or affiliated hospital) has seriously considered the problem, has documented concerns, and has followed the policy arrived at. The issue of informed consent, by printed form, informal notation in the chart, or both, needs also to be considered in this context. Again, no national policy is available, and following local policy or practice is suggested.

Once a patient is started on carbamazepine, a surprising number of patients will show a relative leukopenia with or without a drop in erythrocytes during the first few weeks. Drops to the low 3,000s are not uncommon. If the differential is normal (over 1,000 polymorphonuclear leukocytes) and the patient seems to be benefiting from the treatment, carbamazepine can be continued. After getting a white blood cell count under 3,500, the clinician will almost certainly feel a need to get counts more frequently. The availability of consultation with a friendly, interested, helpful hematologist is an asset to clinicians working with drugs such as carba-mazepine and clozapine.

Carbamazepine also can occasionally cause elevations in liver enzymes, but serious hepatotoxicity is quite rare. It shares with tricyclic antidepressants the ability to slow cardiac conduction. Rashes with carbamazepine are probably a bit more common than with other psychiatric drugs; one recent review estimated a 5% incidence during the initiation of carbamazepine therapy.

Carbamazepine accelerates the metabolism of oral contra-ceptives, corticosteroids, theophylline, warfarin, and halo-peridol. Other drugs—cimetidine, danazol, *d*-propoxyphene, diltiazem, verapamil, isoniazid, and erythromycin—can all raise carbamazepine blood levels. It is hard to judge the clinical importance of these interactions, but increased watch-fulness is in order. We cannot judge the importance of the interaction with birth control pills in terms of their contra-ceptive effectiveness.

Carbamazepine in pregnancy. Until recently, carbamaze-pine was believed to be the safest of the anticonvulsants and the mood stabilizers to use during pregnancy. However, there is a recent report of the occurrence of fetal abnormalities of the type associated with hydantoin—an increased incidence of craniofacial defects, fingernail hypoplasia, and develop-mental delay.

Valproate

In contrast to almost all other drugs used in psychiatry, valproic acid has no rings. (Carbamazepine is tricyclic; valproic acid could be said to be acyclic.) The drug is available in this country in three forms, valproic acid (Depakene), sodium valproate (Depakene syrup), and divalproex sodium (Depa-kote), an enteric-coated stable compound containing both valproic acid and sodium valproate. The amide of valproic acid (Depamide) is used in Europe. All these preparations convert to valproic acid in the plasma. Valproate may be the best general term to encompass all these formulations.

Valproate is approved only for use in simple and complex absence attacks but is probably effective in grand mal and other types of seizures.

Clinical indications.   In an excellent review by McElroy et al. (1987), 20 clinical reports on the use of valproate in psychiatric patients are considered. These involve about 300 patients, but only a handful were treated in placebo-controlled studies. A large multicenter study of valproate versus placebo in mania is nearing completion, but no reports of the results are available.

The early work in the late 1960s by Lambert in France identified valproate as effective in a wide range of manic and schizoaffective manic patients when added to a wide variety of other drugs. Lambert's group reported on over 100 patients but did not describe the patients in any detail. In Lambert's study, in mainly treatment-resistant manic or schizoaffective patients, moderate improvement was reported in over one-half. In patients with acute mania without prior drug therapy, 10 of 14 improved. These results agree with the work of Pope et al. (in press) at McLean Hospital with valproate and with other local clinical experience. Valproate is often a very satisfactory drug in treating mania with clear and substantial improvement occurring within 1–2 weeks at adequate blood levels (over 50 ng/ml).

Valproate may turn out to be particularly useful in rapid cycling bipolar patients and is probably effective as a maintenance therapy in bipolar patients. As with lithium, valproate may do better at preventing future manic episodes than at preventing depressive ones.

The drug's efficacy in chronic schizophrenia without manic features is less clear. Local experience at McLean Hospital is generally disappointing. Occasional depressions may respond, but overall, the drug is not an effective antidepressant.

All of the above statements require a disclaimer. Almost all the reports of good (or bad) response to valproate derive from studies where valproate was added to a wide range of other drugs, particularly lithium and neuroleptics but also antidepressants and carbamazepine. It is hard to be sure whether the other preexisting and concurrent drug therapies contributed to any given patient's success or failure on valproate. None of the available articles suggest that any other psychiatric drug prevents clinical improvement on valproate.

Dosage schedule. The plasma half-life of valproate is on the order of 10–15 hours. Drugs such as carbamazepine, phenobarbital, or phenytoin, given concurrently, will induce hepatic enzymes and shorten valproate's half-life by speeding its metabolism. In contrast to carbamazepine, valproate does not induce its own metabolism. Once an adequate blood level has been attained, it is likely to remain adequate if intake remains constant. Blood levels should be taken about 12 hours after the last dose.

Plasma levels in the range of 50–100 ng/ml are needed for an anticonvulsant effect, although correlations between blood levels and suppression of seizures are only fair to poor in epileptic patients. In manic patients, levels over 50 ng/ml seem to be required for antimanic effect. It is unclear whether much higher levels will work when levels in the 50–70 ng/ml range do not. More side effects are certainly apparent at these higher levels.

In beginning valproate therapy, the enteric-coated divalproex sodium is generally less likely to cause gastrointestinal distress than the other formulations. Initial dosages of 250 mg given two to four times a day are common; the higher daily dose should be reserved for actively manic patients.

Valproic acid plasma levels should be obtained every few days until a level over 50 ng/ml is reached. As with other drugs where dosage is titrated to reach a specified blood level, the final daily dose could be anywhere from 500 to 3,000 mg a day.

Improvement should occur within 2 weeks at a good blood level. If it has not, higher levels could be tried for another 2 weeks, but side effects may prove limiting. Sedation and gastrointestinal distress are the likeliest limiting side effects early in therapy, but only sedation is common and valproate seems generally better tolerated than lithium carbonate.

When a patient improves on valproate, one would originally assume that the drug can be continued at the same dose and level as a maintenance therapy, watching for rare serious toxicity. This may, in fact, be a wise course. However, many patients tried on valproate are already on various other drugs (e.g., lithium, a neuroleptic, carbamazepine, antidepressants, and clonazepam). These drugs can be gradually withdrawn one at a time to determine whether they are needed once valproate is working. Some may prove unnecessary, but tapering and stopping others may invite a relapse. A few patients need two or three mood stabilizers concurrently.

Valproate plus clonazepam is reported to lead to petit mal status. We have never seen this despite the inadvertent use of the combination in a number of patients, but it is a potential problem.

Valproic acid levels can be monitored weekly until stable and presumably adequate levels are achieved, then monthly or less often during prolonged maintenance therapy. The level should be rechecked if new side effects occur or if the clinical condition worsens.

Side effects. The major worry with valproate has been the risk of severe, sometimes fatal, hepatotoxicity. Fatal cases have all been in children under the age of 10, mainly on multiple anticonvulsants. This makes the task of monitoring psychiatric patients on valproate a risk-benefit conundrum. Probably liver function tests should be obtained every month or so just because no one is sure whether severe hepatocellular toxicity will occur. On the other hand, the available data can support the position that liver function tests are unnecessary and that patients and/or relatives should be told of the remote risk and told of early symptoms of liver disease (anorexia, jaundice, nausea, lethargy, etc.). If liver function tests are done, minor elevation in various enzyme levels should not necessarily lead to stopping the drug. One local expert in epilepsy says only elevations in serum bilirubin should be cause for concern. Balancing the apparent clinical benefit to the patient against the abnormality of the liver function tests is reasonable. The better the patient's response, the more one persists in giving valproate in the face of progressively abnormal liver function tests.

Thrombocytopenia and platelet dysfunction have been reported in patients on valproate. Warning patients to report easy bruising or bleeding is indicated. Platelet levels can be checked.

Sedation is the most common side effect of valproate therapy. Tremor can occur, as can ataxia. Weight gain and alopecia can also occur. When valproate is taken during the first trimester of pregnancy, neural tube defects can occur (spina bifida, anencephaly).

Coma and death can occur when valproate is taken with suicidal intent. The drug can be removed by hemodialysis. There is one report that valproate coma was reversed by naloxone.

Clonazepam

Several benzodiazepines, chiefly clonazepam and lorazepam, have been reported to be useful in the treatment of acute mania. Similar reports exist on the efficacy of diazepam in schizophrenic excitements. Of these drugs, clonazepam is somewhat better studied and has been reported to be of some value as an adjunctive medication in the maintenance treatment of bipolar patients.

Chouinard and his associates in Montreal have done essentially all the relevant work with clonazepam in mania. He recommends starting with high doses (e.g., 2 mg three or four times a day) and increasing to 4 mg four times a day in severe or treatment-resistant manic patients. Chouinard finds little sedation with these doses, whereas experience in Boston indicates sedation is more of a problem. Doubters believe clonazepam has no specific antimanic effects and is only a long-acting sedative. The few attempts in our hospitals to treat mania with clonazepam alone have not been successful, with confused sedation occurring with or without persisting mania.

When a bipolar patient in full or partial remission requires a benzodiazepine for sleep or anxiety, clonazepam may be worth trying first in the hope that it has some mood-stabilizing effect. Even if this is not true, clonazepam's long half-life and moderate antiepileptic effect may make it preferable to shorter-acting drugs such as lorazepam or alprazolam.

The side effects of clonazepam are those of all current benzodiazepines: sedation, ataxia, and malcoordination. There are rare patients on any sedative drug who become disinhibited and agitated. Patients with a history of attention-deficit hyperactivity disorder in childhood may be at particular risk for sedative-induced angry agitation. We have seen occasional bipolar patients who thought they felt more angry after taking clonazepam. There are no prospective data on this potential side effect.

Phenytoin

Phenytoin was tried extensively in manic and schizophrenic patients in the 1940s when no better drugs existed. Allowing for the optimism of the time and the absence of blood level determinations, it seems likely that phenytoin is not useful in mania or psychosis.

Phenytoin has been extensively studied in various behavior disorders. Most controlled studies are negative, but there are suggestions that the drug can be useful in patients with angry outbursts or chronic irritability.

Side effects of phenytoin include gum hypertrophy and facial coarsening after prolonged use. Acute side effects are ataxia and confusion.

Drug-Drug Interactions

Because anticonvulsants, when used for primarily psychiatric indications, are most often added to other preexisting drug therapies, clinicians must worry about pharmacokinetic (drug metabolism or blood level) and pharmacodynamic (e.g., two sedative drugs given together produce more sedation than either alone) interactions.

When adding an anticonvulsant to other drugs, it is conventional to measure the anticonvulsant blood level periodically. However, when blood levels of the other psychiatric drugs are meaningful, these should be checked as well to see whether they are raised or lowered significantly. The literature on this issue is very spotty and weak and cannot be relied on to predict what will actually happen when carbamazepine or valproate is added to thioridazine or nortriptyline in a particular patient. This same concern applies, perhaps more markedly, in patients on anticoagulants, digitalis, and cimetidine-like drugs.

Bibliography

Altesman R, Cole JO: Lithium therapy: a practical review, in Psychopharmacology Update. Edited by Cole JO. Lexington, MA, Collamore Press, 1980, pp 3–18

Amdisen A: Lithium and drug interactions. Drugs 24:133–139, 1982

Aronson T, Shukla S, Hirschowitz J, et al: Clonazepam treatment of five lithium-refractory patients with bipolar disorder. Am J Psychiatry 146:77–80, 1989

Ayd F: Carbamazepine for aggression, schizophrenia and nonaffective syndromes. International Drug Therapy Newsletter 19:9–12, 1984

Baestrup P, Schou M: Lithium as a prophylactic agent against recurrent depressions and manic-depressive psychosis. Arch Gen Psychiatry 16:162–172, 1967

Baldessarini RJ, Lipinski JF: Lithium salts: 1970–1975. Ann Intern Med 83:527–533, 1975

Ballenger JC, Post RM: Carbamazepine (Tegretol) in manic-depressive illness: a new treatment. Am J Psychiatry 137:782–790, 1980

Biederman J, Lerner Y, Belmaker RH: Combination of lithium carbonate and haloperidol in schizoaffective disorder. Arch Gen Psychiatry 36:327–333, 1979

Blackwell B: Patient compliance with drug therapy. N Engl J Med 289:249–252, 1973

Cade JF: Lithium salts in treatment of psychotic excitement. Med J Aust 36:349–352, 1949

Carbamazepine update (editorial). Lancet 1:595–596, 1989

Chouinard G, Young S, Annable L: Antimanic effects of clonazepam. Biol Psychiatry 18:451–466, 1983

Cole J, Gardos G, Gelernter J, et al: Lithium carbonate in tardive dyskinesia and schizophrenia, in Tardive Dyskinesia and Affective Disorders. Edited by Gardos G, Casey D. Washington, DC, American Psychiatric Press, 1984, pp 50–73

Cowdry R, Gardner D: Pharmacotherapy of borderline personality disorder: alprazolam, carbamazepine, trifluoperazine and tranylcypromine. Arch Gen Psychiatry 45:111–119, 1988

Davenport Y, Ebert M, Adland M, et al: Couples group therapy as an adjunct to lithium maintenance of the manic patient. Am J Orthopsychiatry 47:495–502, 1977

Davis J: Overview: maintenance therapy in psychiatry, II: affective disorders. Am J Psychiatry 133:1–13, 1976

Deandrea D, Walker D, Mehlmauer M, et al: Dermatological reactions to lithium: a critical review of the literature. J Clin Psychopharmacol 2:199–204, 1982

Delva N, Letemendia F: Lithium treatment in schizophrenia and schizoaffective disorders. Br J Psychiatry 141:387–400, 1982

DePaulo JR Jr, Correa EI, Sapir DG: Renal glomerular function and long-term lithium therapy. Am J Psychiatry 138:324–327, 1981

Dorns W, Ostrow DG, Anton R, et al: Lithium treatment of depressed and nondepressed alcoholics. JAMA 262:1646–1652, 1989

Emrich H, Okuma T, Muller A (eds): Anticonvulsants in Affective Disorders (Excerpta Medica International Congress Series No 626). Amsterdam, Excerpta Medica, 1984

Evans RW, Gualtiere T: Carbamazepine: a neuropsychological and psychiatric profile. Clin Neuropharmacol 8:221–241, 1985

Fawcett J, Clark DC, Aagesen CA, et al: A double-blind, placebo-controlled trial of lithium carbonate therapy for alcoholism. Arch Gen Psychiatry 44:248–256, 1987

Frankenburg FR, Tohen M, Cohen BM, et al: Long-term response to carbamazepine: a retrospective review. J Clin Psychopharmacol 8:130–132, 1988

Gardner E: Long-term preventive care in depression: the use of bupropion in patients intolerant of other antidepressants. J Clin Psychiatry 44:163–169, 1983

Gelenberg AJ, Carroll JA, Baudhuin MG, et al: The meaning of serum lithium levels in maintenance therapy of mood disorders: a review of the literature. J Clin Psychiatry 50 (suppl 12):17–22, 1989

Gelenberg AJ, Kane JM, Keller MB, et al: Comparison of standard and low serum levels of lithium for maintenance treatment of bipolar disorder. N Engl J Med 321:1489–1493, 1989

Groff P: Long term lithium treatment and the kidney. Can J Psychiatry 25:535–541, 1980

Himmelhoch JM, Forest J, Neil JF, et al: Thiazide-lithium synergy in refractory mood swings. Am J Psychiatry 134:149–152, 1977

Himmelhoch JM, Poust RI, Mallinger AG: Adjustment of lithium dose during lithium-chlorothiazide therapy. Clin Pharmacol Ther 22:225–227, 1977

Jefferson JW, Greist JH: Primer of Lithium Therapy. Baltimore, MD, Williams & Wilkins, 1977

Jefferson JW, Greist JH, Baudhuin M: Lithium: interactions with other drugs. J Clin Psychopharmacol 1:124–134, 1981

Jefferson JW, Greist JH, Ackerman DL, et al: Lithium Encyclopedia for Clinical Practice, 2nd Edition. Washington, DC, American Psychiatric Press, 1986

Jeste D, Wyatt R: Therapeutic strategies against tardive dyskinesia. Arch Gen Psychiatry 39:803–816, 1982

Joffe R, Post R, Roy-Byrne P, et al: Hematological effects of carbamazepine in patients with affective illness. Am J Psychiatry 142:1196–1199, 1985

Jones K, Lacro R, Johnson K, et al: Pattern of malformations in the children of women treated with carbamazepine during pregnancy. N Engl J Med 320:1161–1666, 1989

Kishimoto A, Ogura C, Hazama H, et al: Long-term prophylactic effects of carbamazepine in affective disorder. Br J Psychiatry 143:327–331, 1983

Klein DF, Gittelman R, Quitkin F, et al: Diagnosis and Treatment of Psychiatric Disorders: Adults and Children, 2nd Edition. Baltimore, MD, Williams & Wilkins, 1980

Klein E, Bental E, Lerer B, et al: Carbamazepine and haloperidol v placebo and haloperidol in excited psychoses. Arch Gen Psychiatry 41:165–170, 1984

Kline NS, Wren JC, Cooper TB, et al: Evaluation of lithium therapy in chronic and periodic alcoholism. Am J Med Sci 268:15–22, 1974

Kripke D, Robinson D: Ten years with a lithium group. McLean Hospital Journal 10:l-ll, 1985

Lambert P, Carraz G, Borselli S, et al: Dipropylacetamide in the treatment of manic-depressive psychosis. L'Encephale l:25–31, 1975

Lipinski JF, Pope HD Jr: Possible synergistic action between carbamazepine and lithium carbonate in the treatment of three acutely manic patients. Am J Psychiatry 139:948–949, 1982

McElroy SL, Pope HG Jr (eds): Use of Anticonvulsants in Psychiatry: Recent Advances. Clifton, NJ, Oxford Health Care, 1988

McElroy SL, Keck PE Jr, Pope HG Jr: Sodium valproate: its use in primary psychiatric disorders. J Clin Psychopharmacol 7:16–24, 1987

Mendels J: Lithium in the treatment of depression. Am J Psychiatry 133:373–378, 1976

Merry J, Reynolds CM, Bailey J, et al: Prophylactic treatment of alcoholism by lithium carbonate. Lancet 2:481–482, 1976

Modell J, Lenox R, Weiner S: Inpatient clinical trial of lorazepam for the management of manic agitation. J Clin Psychopharmacol 5:109–113, 1985

Nierenberg AA, Price LH, Charney DS, et al: After lithium augmentation: a retrospective follow-up of patients with antidepressant-refractory depression. J Affective Disord 18:167–175, 1990

Ortiz A, Dabbagh M, Gershon G: Lithium: clinical use, toxicology and mode of action, in Clinical Psychopharmacology, 2nd Edition. Edited by Bernstein J. Littleton, MA, Wright PSG, 1984, pp 111–144

Post RM, Uhde TW: Carbamazepine in bipolar illness. Psychopharmacol Bull 21:10–17, 1985

Post RM, Rubinow DR, Ballenger JC: Conditioning and sensitisation in the longitudinal course of affective illness. Br J Psychiatry 149:191–201, 1986

Post R, Uhde T, Roy-Byrne P, et al: Correlates of antimanic response to carbamazepine. Psychiatry Res 21:71–83, 1987

Prien R: Long-term prophylactic pharmacologic treatment of bipolar illness, in Psychiatry Update: The American Psychiatric Association Annual Review, Vol 2. Edited by Grinspoon L. Washington, DC, American Psychiatric Press, 1983, pp 303–318

Prien RF, Caffey EM Jr: Long-term maintenance drug therapy in recurrent affective illness: current status and issues. Diseases of the Nervous System 38:981–992, 1977

Prien R, Caffey E, Klett C: A comparison of lithium carbonate and chlorpromazine in the treatment of excited schizoaffectives. Arch Gen Psychiatry 27:182–189, 1972

Prien R, Caffey E, Klett C: A comparison of lithium carbonate and chlorpromazine in the treatment of mania. Arch Gen Psychiatry 26:146–153, 1972

Prien R, Kupfer D, Mansky P, et al: Drug therapy in the prevention of recurrences in unipolar and bipolar affective disorders. Arch Gen Psychiatry 41:1096–1104, 1984

Quitkin F, Rifkin A, Klein DF, et al: Prophylaxis in unipolar affective disorder. Am J Psychiatry 133:1091–1092, 1976

Ramsey TA, Cox M: Lithium and the kidney. Am J Psychiatry 139:443–449, 1982

Rifkin A, Quitkin F, Carrillo C, et al: Lithium carbonate in emotionally unstable character disorder. Arch Gen Psychiatry 28:519–523, 1972

Rosenbaum JF (ed): New uses of clonazepam in psychiatry. J Clin Psychiatry 48:3S–56S, 1987

Sachs G, Rosenbaum J, Jones L: Adjunctive clonazepam for maintenance treatment of bipolar affective disorder. J Clin Psychopharmacol 10:42–47, 1990

Schou M: The range of clinical uses of lithium, in Lithium in Medical Practice. Edited by Johnson FN, Johnson S. Baltimore, MD, University Park Press, 1978

Schou M: Artistic productivity and lithium prophylaxis in manic-depressive illness. Br J Psychiatry 135:97–103, 1979

Schou M: Lithium prophylaxis: myths and realities. Am J Psychiatry 146:573–576, 1989

Sheard JH, Marini JL, Bridges CI, et al: The effect of lithium on impulsive aggressive behavior in man. Am J Psychiatry 133:1409–1413, 1976

Shopsin B: Bupropion's prophylactic efficacy in bipolar affective illness. J Clin Psychiatry 44:163–169, 1983

Teicher M, Altesman R, Cole J, et al: Possible nephrotoxic interaction of lithium and metronidazole. JAMA 254:3365–3366, 1987

Teratogenic effects of carbamazepine (letter to the editor). N Engl J Med 321:1480–1481, 1989

Tilkian AG, Schroder JS, Kao JJ, et al: The cardiovascular effects of lithium in man. Am J Med 61:665–670, 1976

Tupin J: Management of violent patients, in Manual of Psychiatric Therapeutics. Edited by Shader R. Boston, MA, Little, Brown, 1975, pp 125–133

Uhde T, Post R, Ballenger J, et al: Carbamazepine in the treatment of neuropsychiatric disorders, in Anticonvulsants in Affective Disorders (Excerpta Medica International Congress Series No 626). Edited by Emrich H, Okuma T, Muller A. Amsterdam, Excerpta Medica, 1984, pp 111–131

Vendsborg PB, Bech P, Rafaelson OJ: Lithium treatment and weight gain. Acta Psychiatr Scand 53:139–147, 1976

Yorkston N, Zaki S, Harvard C: Some practical aspects of using propranolol in the treatment of schizophrenia, in Propranolol and Schizophrenia. Edited by Roberts E, Amacher P. New York, Alan R Liss, 1978, pp 83–97

Antianxiety Agents

6

Anxiolytic agents are the most commonly used psychotropic drugs. The vast majority of prescriptions for these medications are issued by internists, family practitioners, and obstetricians. Psychiatrists write less than 20% of the prescriptions for anxiolytics in this country, reflecting, in part, the fact that most anxious patients never see psychiatrists. Moreover, anxiolytics are prescribed for many varieties of patients who do not suffer from a primary anxiety disorder. Rather, they are prescribed for patients who present to primary-care physicians with somatic complaints or true somatic disease.

Antianxiety agents may be divided into many subclasses, of which the benzodiazepines are the most frequently prescribed. Several of the subclasses of anxiolytics (e.g., benzodiazepines) include agents that are marketed primarily as hypnotics (e.g., flurazepam). The differentiation between anxiolytic and hypnotic benzodiazepines is somewhat artifactual, with most of the traditional anxiolytic agents enjoying sedative properties (e.g., diazepam) . In this manual we have separated the pharmacologic treatments of anxiety from those of insomnia—albeit somewhat artificially—since almost any sedative or antianxiety drug can be used at a low dose in the daytime for anxiety and at a high dose for difficulty in sleeping.

The first major anxiolytic group, the barbiturates, were developed as sedative-hypnotic and antiepileptic agents and were first introduced in the early 1900s. These drugs are also discussed extensively in the chapter on hypnotics (Chapter 7). Meprobamate was introduced almost 60 years later as a sedative-anxiolytic agent. Although the use of these two classes has waned in recent years, they are still more commonly prescribed than one might imagine; meprobamate and phenobarbital represent approximately 7% of the anxiolytic market. Benzodiazepines, introduced in the early 1960s, dramatically changed the pharmacologic approach to anxiety. First developed as muscle relaxants, their anxiolytic-hypnotic properties and wider safety margin in overdosage and addictive potential quickly became apparent. These drugs now account for over 90% of the anxiolytic market. Buspirone, a serotonin agonist with some mixed dopamine effects, was released for use in anxiety in the United States in 1987.

Less widely used pharmacologic approaches to anxiety include antihistamines and autonomic agents (e.g., beta-blockers). The former act primarily via a general sedative action; the latter—which are being used increasingly—act by blocking peripheral or central noradrenergic activity and many of the manifestations of anxiety (tremor, palpitations, sweating, etc.). Several of the phenothiazines also have indications in anxiety, although in the United States they have become less widely used in recent years for this purpose. Several antidepressants appear effective in both generalized anxiety disorder and panic disorder, and clomipramine, now available in the United States, has been reported to be very effective in some patients with obsessive-compulsive disorder. A number of specific serotonin reuptake blockers (e.g., fluvoxamine and fluoxetine) are being intensively studied as treatments for obsessive-compulsive disorder.

BENZODIAZEPINES

Indications

In addition to anxiety, benzodiazepines are indicated for muscle relaxation, insomnia, status epilepticus (diazepam), myoclonic epilepsy (clonazepam), preoperative anesthesia, and alcohol withdrawal. One new member—the triazolobenzodiazepine alprazolam—is also indicated for anxiety associated with depression (as is lorazepam), and recent studies have indicated alprazolam may also parallel imipramine and phenelzine in having both antipanic and antidepressant properties (see Chapter 3). Another triazolobenzodiazepine, adinazolam, appears to also enjoy antidepressant and antipanic properties (see Chapter 3). This compound had not been released as of this writing. Clonazepam has also recently been shown to have some antipanic effects.

Mode of Action

In recent years, considerable attention has been paid to the potential mode of action of benzodiazepines, spurred on by the identification of specific receptor sites. These sites, found in various brain regions, are coupled to gamma-aminobutyric acid (GABA) receptors. This receptor complex appears to mediate the anxiolytic, sedative, and anticonvulsant actions of the benzodiazepines. The location of specific receptors may be related to the relative anticonvulsant, anxiolytic, or sedative properties of the various benzodiazepines. Some pharmacologists have hypothesized that it may be possible to develop new compounds that either bind more specifically to certain receptors or that act as partial agonists to produce anxiolysis without sedation. These approaches are being actively explored, but we do not anticipate that such drugs will be available in the near term. In addition, such drugs may substantially reduce the risk for tolerance, dependence, and withdrawal effects.

The triazolobenzodiazepine alprazolam also appears to have effects on noradrenergic systems, causing downregulation of postsynaptic beta-receptors in reserpine-treated mice and increasing the activity of the N-protein in humans (the protein that couples the postsynaptic receptor to the intraneuronal energy system). These effects may help to explain the drug's antipanic and moderate antidepressant effects.

Adinazolam appears to enjoy more pronounced effects on noradrenergic and probably serotonergic systems than does alprazolam (see Chapter 3). These (and probably other) benzodiazepines may also exert downregulating effects on corticotropin-releasing factor (CRF), a peptide that both initiates the hypothalamic-pituitary-adrenal (HPA) axis stress response and may affect central catecholamine systems as well. Thus, some benzodiazepines exert extremely complicated neurochemical effects.

Subclasses

The anxiolytic benzodiazepines are commonly divided into three subclasses on the basis of structure: 2-keto (chlordiazepoxide, diazepam, prazepam, clorazepate, halazepam, clonazepam, and the hypnotic flurazepam); 3-hydroxy (oxazepam, lorazepam, and the hypnotic temazepam); and triazolo (alprazolam, adinazolam, and the hypnotic triazolam) (see Figure 6-1 and Table 6-1). The pharmacokinetic properties (i.e., half-lives) vary among these classes, in part reflecting differences in their modes of drug metabolism, as summarized in Table 6-2. The 2-keto drugs and their active metabolites are oxidized in the liver, and, since this process

2-KETO-LIKE

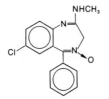

Chlordiazepoxide

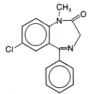

Diazepam

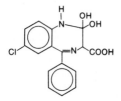

Clorazepate

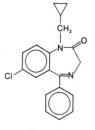

Prazepam

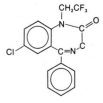

Halazepam

3-HYDROXY

TRIAZOLO

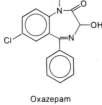

Oxazepam

Lorazepam

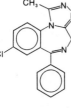

Alprazolam

Figure 6-1. Chemical structures of anxiolytic benzodiazepines.

is relatively slow, these compounds have relatively long half-lives. For example, the half-life of diazepam is approximately 40 hours. One active metabolite (desmethyldiazepam) has an even longer half-life—about 60 hours. Moreover, since desmethyldiazepam is further metabolized to oxazepam, which is also active as an anxiolytic (Table 6-1), diazepam imparts

Table 6-1. Benzodiazepines: specific compounds, available preparations, and anxiolytic dosage ranges

Generic name	Brand name	Dosage forms	Dosage range (mg/day)*
2-Keto-			
chlordiazepoxide†	Librium	Capsule: 5, 10, 25 mg; Ampule: 20 mg/ml (5-ml ampule)	15–40; 50–100 once (2.5–50 tid)
	Libritabs	Tablet: 5, 10, 25 mg	15–40
clorazepate†	Tranxene	Tablet: 3.75, 7.5, 15 mg; Capsule: 3.75, 7.5, 15 mg	15–60
	Tranxene SD	Tablet: 11.25, 22.5 mg	11.25–45
diazepam†	Valium	Tablet: 2, 5, 10 mg; Parenteral: 5 mg/ml (2-ml syringe) (2-ml ampule) (10-ml vial)	5–40
	Diazepam Oral (liquid)	5 mg/5 ml, 10 mg/10 ml	
	Valrelease	Capsule: 15 mg (slow release)	15–30
halazepam	Paxipam	Tablet: 20, 40 mg	60–160
prazepam†	Centrax	Tablet: 5, 10 mg	20–60
3-Hydroxy-			
lorazepam†	Ativan	Tablet: 0.5, 1, 2 mg; Parenteral: 2, 4 mg/ml (1- and 10-ml vials), 2-ml syringe	1–6; 1–2
oxazepam†	Serax	Tablet: 15 mg; Capsule: 10, 15, 30 mg	45–120
Triazolo-			
alprazolam	Xanax	Tablet: 0.25, 0.5, 1 mg	1–4

* Approximate dosage ranges. Some patients will require higher dosages; others may respond to dosages below the range.
† Available in generic form.

Table 6-2. Benzodiazepines: absorption and pharmacokinetics

Generic name	Oral absorption	Major active components	Approximate half-life (hours)*
2-Keto-			
chlordiazepoxide	intermediate	chlordiazepoxide	20
		desmethylchlordiazepoxide	30
		demoxepam	Unknown
		desmethyldiazepam	60
clorazepate	fast	desmethyldiazepam	60
diazepam	fast	diazepam	40
		desmethyldiazepam	60
halazepam	slow	desmethyldiazepam	60
prazepam	slow	desmethyldiazepam	60
3-Hydroxy-			
lorazepam	intermediate	lorazepam	14
oxazepam	slow to intermediate	oxazepam	9
Triazolo-			
alprazolam	intermediate	alprazolam	14

* Based on ranges of half-lives reported in healthy, young normal volunteers.

long-range sedative and anxiolytic effects. The half-life of clonazepam is approximately 40 hours.

Many of the marketed 2-keto drugs are prodrugs—they are themselves inactive but eventually form active metabolites. Thus prazepam, clorazepate, and halazepam are mere precursors for desmethyldiazepam—as is diazepam. Differences among these specific 2-keto compounds revolve around the rates of absorption and the specific active metabolites formed.

In contrast, the 3-hydroxy compounds are metabolized via direct conjugation with a glucuronide radical, a process that is more rapid than oxidation and does not involve the formation of active metabolites. The two major examples of this subclass are oxazepam and lorazepam, which have considerably shorter half-lives (9 and 14 hours, respectively) than do their 2-keto counterparts. Similarly, the hypnotic temazepam has a half-life (8 hours) that is much shorter than flurazepam's.

The triazolo compounds are also oxidized; however, they appear to have more limited active metabolites and thus relatively shorter half-lives. The half-life of alprazolam is about 14 hours; adinazolam, 2 hours; and N-desmethyladinazolam (its active metabolite), 4 hours; that of the hypnotic triazolam is 3–4 hours. A sustained-relief form of adinazolam is currently under active investigation.

The pharmacokinetic properties of benzodiazepines that are oxidized in the liver may be affected by other medications. Of particular note, cimetidine (Tagamet) and birth control pills inhibit liver oxidative enzymes and thus slow the degradation of the 2-keto and triazolo compounds. Clinicians should keep this in mind in treating anxious patients who are also taking these nonpsychotropic drugs.

Other differences among benzodiazepines revolve around their rates of absorption and distribution. For example, although prazepam and clorazepate are similar in structure and both are prodrugs of desmethyldiazepam, the two differ in terms of the metabolic processes required for absorption and thus in the rates at which they appear in blood (Table 6-2). Clorazepate and diazepam are rapidly absorbed and produce peaks in plasma levels more quickly than does prazepam, whose absorption is mediated via slower processes. Halazepam's conversion to desmethyldiazepam is even slower.

The lipophilic and hydrophilic properties of these drugs also vary, resulting in pronounced differences in how quickly they work and for how long. Drugs that are more lipophilic (e.g., diazepam) will enter the brain more quickly—"turning on" the effect promptly, but "turning off" more quickly as well—as they disappear into body fat. Less lipophilic compounds (e.g., lorazepam) will produce clinical effects more slowly but may provide more sustained relief. These properties are largely independent of pharmacokinetics. Some drugs with long half-lives (e.g., diazepam) can also be highly lipophilic, providing rapid relief but for shorter periods than one might predict from half-life data alone. In contrast, lorazepam is less lipophilic and turns on and off more slowly, potentially providing more sustained effects, despite its shorter half-life compared with diazepam. In short, traditional half-life pharmacokinetics can be misleading and only tell a part of the story of how drugs work.

In addition, investigators have begun to pay more attention to relative receptor affinity, a property that may play a more important role in determining the duration of action than previously thought. High-potency benzodiazepines, such as lorazepam and alprazolam, may have such high affinity that withdrawal symptoms may be far more intense than one might expect from inspecting other variables such as half-lives. Interestingly, oxazepam, which is similar in lipid solubility and half-life to lorazepam, appears to produce less in the way of withdrawal symptoms. This position has been most eloquently stated by Lader in the United Kingdom. Unfortunately, there are few data to confirm or refute this assertion.

Although several of the benzodiazepines are available for

parenteral usage (see Table 6-1), there is wide variability in the absorption properties of these compounds when given intramuscularly. For example, lorazepam is relatively rapidly absorbed when given intramuscularly. In contrast, chlordiazepoxide and diazepam are slowly absorbed. Lorazepam has become increasingly popular as an adjunctive treatment for agitation in acutely psychotic patients and also appears to relieve catatonic and depressive stupor. Oral concentrate forms of benzodiazepines, except for oral diazepam solution (with which we have no experience), are not available in the United States.

Dosage Ranges

The efficacy of benzodiazepines in patients with symptomatic anxiety or diagnosable anxiety disorders has been established in double-blind, random assignment comparisons with placebo. When treating a patient with generalized anxiety disorder, the clinician should begin at approximately 2 mg tid of diazepam with increases as needed to a maximum regular daily dose of diazepam of 40 mg. A modal dose of diazepam for generalized anxiety disorder is 15–20 mg/day. Chlordiazepoxide has a much wider dosage range. Recommended starting dose is 5–10 mg po tid with a maximum of 60 mg/day for anxiety. The dosage of chlordiazepoxide used for acute alcohol withdrawal is much higher—50–200 mg/day. Generally, clinicians prescribe 25 mg every 1–2 hours until symptomatic relief or sedation occurs, up to a maximum of 200 mg/day. Dosage ranges of the anxiolytic benzodiazepines are listed in Table 6-1.

The use of alprazolam in panic patients may require higher dosages than those used in generalized anxiety disorder. Currently, alprazolam is approved in dosages up to 4 mg/day; however, some studies on panic disorder or depression have used doses of up to 10 mg/day. In our early studies on depression, we used the much higher dosage regimen, but we have been impressed that patients generally do not require more than 4 mg/day to respond and some are even oversedated at 2–3 mg/day. Because of the concern about dependence, this drug should be used at the lowest effective dose possible. Starting dosage of alprazolam in both generalized anxiety disorder and panic disorder should be 1.5 mg/day or less given in divided doses, with a gradual increase in dosage as tolerated by the patient. In treating patients with panic disorder, alprazolam dosage should be increased to not only block panic attacks but anticipatory anxiety as well. This often requires higher dosages (4–5 mg) in the first 6 + weeks. Over time, however, as patients overcome their anticipatory anxiety, the dosage can be reduced to 2–3 mg for continued blocking of panic attacks. Although alprazolam was thought to have unique antipanic properties, recent reports indicate that lorazepam, clonazepam, and diazepam may all be effective in ameliorating or preventing panic symptoms. Clonazepam is used in 1- to 3-mg doses per day.

In patients who have occasional bouts of moderate anxiety ocurring only every few days or weeks, benzodiazepines are best used as prn medication. Diazepam's ability to act rapidly without prolonged sedation makes it particularly useful in such situations in patients not prone to drug abuse. Other benzodiazepines can also be used in this manner, of course. Oxazepam's slow absorption rate raises concern about its utility as a prn medication. However, patient acceptance of this drug is fairly good, and oxazepam's low abuse liability makes it a reasonable choice in some patients.

One major area of debate revolves around how long to use these drugs for patients with significant anxiety. For those patients whose anxiety is very acute and related to specific stressors, use of these agents should be directed at reduction of acute symptoms, and thus prolonged use beyond 1–2 weeks is generally not required or advised. In patients whose anxiety symptoms are of a month's duration (i.e., DSM-III generalized anxiety disorder), we recommend treatment for 3–4 weeks at doses that provide relief, then reduction of dosage to the minimum needed for maintenance for the next 1–2 months, and then discontinuation when possible. Patients who meet DSM-III-R criteria for generalized anxiety disorder will by definition be more chronic and will require longer treatment (e.g., 4–6 months or longer) before attempting discontinuation.

Unfortunately, there are many patients who obtain relief from these drugs but who relapse when they are stopped. Further, since many patients seem to do well on reasonable dosages over longer periods, the clinician may be faced with a difficult decision of how long to maintain the benzodiazepine. This dilemma is intensified by the observations that tolerance can develop to benzodiazepines, suggesting to some that the apparent relief experienced by patients reflects a nonspecific psychological effect.

Although tolerance can occur, it is our belief that some patients actually do not develop tolerance but are still responding. We base this observation on the numbers of patients we have seen over the years who have functioned well on a given daily dose of benzodiazepine and have not found themselves escalating their total daily intake. Recent longer-term data from alprazolam studies indicate that panic patients do not escalate their daily dosages but, rather, frequently lower them over time. There does not appear to be a loss of efficacy of alprazolam in patients followed for up to 1 year. It is our impression that animal and human models of tolerance may not be totally applicable to chronic anxiety per se; rather, such models emphasize self-administration of drug or drug-induced ataxia produced in "normal" specimens but do not take into full account the biological and clinical status of the anxious patient. If possible, the clinician should attempt to taper the patient off benzodiazepines, using psychotherapy or behavior therapy to help patients deal with their anxiety. Some patients, however, may require continued pharmacologic intervention.

True longer-term harmful effects of benzodiazepines have not been convincingly described. For example, Lader (1982) reported computed tomographic scan abnormalities in a series of patients who had taken benzodiazepines on a long-term basis. Although these observations could be interpreted as indicating that these drugs produce organic/structural changes in brain tissue (as chronic alcohol use does), an equally acceptable explanation is that some anxious patients who require chronic treatment with benzodiazepines may have neuropsychiatric disorders as evidenced by computed tomographic scan abnormalities. A study by Lucki et al. (1986) of patients on chronic long-term benzodiazepine treatment failed to show significant cognitive impairment on psychometric tests. However, some investigators believe such impairment can occur, particularly in the elderly.

Are these drugs addictive? Do they produce withdrawal symptoms? Studies in animals indicate that benzodiazepines can reinforce use and can produce physical dependence and tolerance. Available survey and treatment facility data suggest that benzodiazepines are rarely sought after or craved in the sense that heroin or cocaine are. They are used to modulate the effects of primary drugs of abuse (e.g., cocaine) or as backup drugs when more euphoriant drugs are not available as part of a polysubstance abuse problem.

Risk factors for benzodiazepine abuse include a history of alcohol or other substance abuse and the presence of a personality disorder. In patients with a history of substance abuse, benzodiazepines should generally not be prescribed. In patients with an Axis II disorder, they should be administered only if necessary and for brief periods at low dosages. Benzodiazepine dependence is mainly, or at least partially, an iatrogenic problem in that patients receive the medication from physicians for originally legitimate reasons but then take it for too long or in too large dosages. Possible length of treatment with these drugs should be thought out in advance of their prescription and longer-term trials should be monitored carefully.

Should one withdraw patients who have taken benzodiazepines regularly over longer periods? As a rule, this is sensible, reducing at a maximum rate of approximately 10% per day. In their classic study of benzodiazepine withdrawal, Rickels et al. (1983) noted that patients who had been on benzodiazepines for more than 8 months more frequently (43%) demonstrated withdrawal symptoms on abrupt discontinuation under double-blind conditions than did patients who were taking benzodiazepines for shorter periods (5%). In a more recent study, this group reported similar rates of withdrawal symptoms in patients who had been maintained on clorazepate for 6 months (Rickels et al. 1988). Patients did not experience withdrawal symptoms when they were discontinued from buspirone. Pecknold et al. (1988) reported that sudden discontinuation after an 8-week trial of alprazolam resulted in symptoms of anxiety in some 35% of panic patients. Some of these patients may have experienced re-emergence of their panic symptoms rather than withdrawal.

Common withdrawal symptoms include jitteriness, anxiety, palpitations, clamminess, sweating, nausea, confusion, and heightened sensitivity to light and sound. Seizures represent the most worrisome of withdrawal reactions but fortunately are generally rare. No patients in the 1983 study by Rickels et al. experienced seizures. Seizures with abrupt diazepam withdrawal occur some 5–7 days after stopping the drug and not within 24 hours, reflecting the long half-lives of diazepam and desmethyldiazepam. With shorter-acting drugs (e.g., lorazepam and alprazolam), withdrawal symptoms emerge more rapidly—within 2–3 days. Thus with diazepam, physicians cannot be confident that seizures will not occur unless the patient has been off the drug at least 1 week. Any signs of withdrawal (even at day 5) should be reviewed carefully, and consideration should be given to reinstituting the drug and then withdrawing it more gradually.

A few days after discontinuation of benzodiazepines, some patients reexperience their original anxiety symptoms but in a more severe form—so-called rebound anxiety. (In the case of hypnotics, this takes the form of rebound insomnia.) This syndrome is generally transient, lasting up to 48–72 hours.

The widespread use of the potent benzodiazepine alprazolam has led to concern whether it is more difficult to discontinue treatment with this drug than with other benzodiazepines. No data indicate that this is the case, although alprazolam discontinuation can be difficult in some patients.

When discontinuing patients from an alprazolam dosage of 4–5 mg/day, a gradual dosage reduction of 0.5 mg every 7 days to 2 mg/day appears reasonable. Clinical data suggest some patients cannot tolerate this rate of reduction, particularly when daily dosages are at or below 2 mg/day. At 2 mg/day or less, reduction by 0.25 mg every 7 days is reasonable.

Some patients experience withdrawal symptoms (or re-emerging panic or other anxiety) even when using a conservative dose-reduction strategy. For these patients, switching to clonazepam—a longer-acting benzodiazepine—can be helpful (Herman et al. 1987). The strategy calls for prescribing clonazepam at approximately one-half the dose of alprazolam, with patients using small doses of alprazolam as needed for the first few days. Clonazepam dose is adjusted upward depending on the amount of alprazolam used. Patients can then be maintained on clonazepam, which can later be discontinued. Although this strategy is frequently effective, a number of caveats should be raised. Some patients find clonazepam to be more sedating than alprazolam and do not tolerate the switch easily. Another caveat is that some patients may find it difficult to withdraw from clonazepam.

Another strategy is to add carbamazepine to the benzodiazepine and to stabilize the dosage to produce plasma levels in the 4–8 mg/L range. After stabilizing the anticonvulsant, the benzodiazepine can be discontinued. We have used this strategy with some success, although the anticonvulsant often does not block all withdrawal symptoms.

A final strategy is to start the patient on a tricyclic antidepressant (TCA) while he or she continues to take a benzodiazepine. This can help to block reemerging panic attacks on benzodiazepine discontinuation. After stabilizing the TCA dose, benzodiazepine discontinuation can proceed as above.

Gradual dosage reduction of a shorter-acting benzodiaze-pine is difficult for some patients, either because of the physical or the psychological effects produced. In such pa-tients, hospitalization and the application of more aggressive discontinuation protocols that employ barbiturates are war-ranted (see Chapter 11).

Side Effects

Compared with many other classes of psychotropic agents, benzodiazepines enjoy relatively favorable side effect profiles. The most common side effect is sedation, which is in part dose related and can be managed by reducing dosage. Other effects include dizziness, weakness, ataxia, anterograde am-nesia (particularly with the short-acting benzodiazepines, e.g., triazolam), decreased motoric performance (e.g., driv-ing), nausea, and slight hypotension. Falls in elderly patients have been reported to be related to use of longer-acting benzodiazepines (see Chapter 12). In the popular press, there have been reports of severe dyscontrol syndromes on certain benzodiazepines, particularly triazolam (see Chapter 7). We personally have not encountered any in our clinical practice. Fortunately, these drugs have a relatively wide safety margin, and deaths due to benzodiazepine ingestion alone are rare. Most deaths that have involved these drugs have also been associated with concomitant ingestion of other agents—e.g., alcohol or tricyclic antidepressants.

BARBITURATES

Thirty to forty years ago, the only medications widely used in psychiatric patients for the treatment of anxiety or agitation were barbiturates. Longer-acting barbiturates, such as phenobarbital or barbital, were widely used for daytime sedation, and shorter-acting barbiturates with, presumably, more rapid onset of action, such as secobarbital, amobarbital, or pentobarbital, were widely used as hypnotics. (For further discussion of hypnotics, see Chapter 7.) Amobarbital in particular was also widely used as a daytime sedative and, in combination with *d*-amphetamine, as a widely used mixed sedative and stimulant called Dexamyl, no longer available in the United States. Phenobarbital is the only barbiturate that is widely used in general clinical practice at the present time, and it is used essentially only in the treatment of epilepsy. It has some efficacy as a daytime sedative and possibly as an antianxiety agent in doses of 15–30 mg three or four times a day. It is also used as a long-acting sedative (the "methadone" of the barbiturate group) in some detoxification programs in withdrawing patients from shorter-acting sedatives or occasionally from alcohol.

In double-blind controlled clinical trials comparing phenobarbital with placebo and a benzodiazepine or meprobamate, phenobarbital was generally slightly more effective than placebo and inferior to the newer antianxiety agents. In many such studies the dose of phenobarbital used was fixed and low, and its efficacy may well have been played down by the conditions of the trial. However, many patients find the sedative effect of phenobarbital rather dysphoric and unpleasant, and its utility as an antianxiety drug is therefore limited. In patients taking phenobarbital for epilepsy and, more strikingly, in children or even adults with a history of

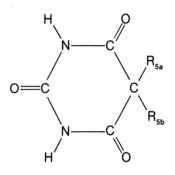

Compound	R_{5a}	R_{5b}
Amobarbital	ethyl	isopentyl
Aprobarbital	allyl	isopropyl
Butabarbital	ethyl	sec-butyl
Pentobarbital	ethyl	l-methylbutyl
Phenobarbital	ethyl	phenyl
Secobarbital	allyl	l-methylbutyl

Figure 6-2. General chemical formulas of the barbiturates.

attention-deficit disorder, phenobarbital can in fact aggravate hyperactivity and disorganized behavior. Occasionally, increased hyperactivity and disturbed behavior in some children and adolescents can be traced to antiasthmatics that contain phenobarbital.

On the other hand, it is quite possible that amobarbital or other relatively shorter-acting barbiturates might be as effective as benzodiazepines in the daytime treatment of anxiety. Several enjoy indications for daytime sedation, and of these butabarbital (Butisol) is occasionally used in such a way. (See Table 6-3 for preparations and Figure 6-2 for structures of the barbiturates.) No good controlled clinical trials have been done comparing such shorter-acting and possibly less dysphoric and more euphoric barbiturates with benzodiazepines. There is, however, little point in carrying out such trials, since it is reasonably clear that the addiction and abuse liability of barbiturates is substantially greater than that of most benzodiazepines, even including diazepam. The barbiturates like amobarbital also have the disadvantage of the lethal dose being relatively low, perhaps 1,000 mg taken in a single overdose. In addition, barbiturates induce enzymes that metabolize other important medications. It is also possible but not proven that tolerance develops somewhat more rapidly to the barbiturates when taken in escalating dosages. In a classic study by Isbell et al. (1950), performed at the Addiction Research Center in Lexington in the 1940s, patients on very large daily doses of barbiturates managed to complain of going into withdrawal while being so ataxic and malcoordinated that they were falling down when they tried to walk and were slurring their speech. This suggests that the tolerance to the antianxiety and/or euphoriant effects of the barbiturates develops more rapidly than does tolerance to the drugs' effects on psychomotor functions. Very large doses of benzodiazepines taken chronically do not appear to have this property.

Amobarbital sodium (Amytal) as a parenteral solution is still of some value in psychiatry. When given intramuscularly to quiet agitated behavior in disturbed or psychotic patients, a dose of 100 mg is common with a range between 50 and 250 mg, based on the weight of the patient and the degree of excitement. It has one major advantage over parenteral antipsychotics such as chlorpromazine, haloperidol, or loxapine in that it acts more rapidly, perhaps in 10–20 minutes, and when it acts, it tends to produce sleep rather than tranquilization. We know of no systematic study of the relative utility of amobarbital compared with either haloperidol or chlorpromazine in the treatment of acutely disturbed behavior requiring only a single injection. The advantage of amobarbital as noted is that it produces sleep relatively rapidly. The disadvantage is that when the patient awakens, there is no residual antipsychotic activity to modulate the

Table 6-3. Other antianxiety/daytime sedative agents

Generic name	Brand name	Dosage forms	Dosage range (mg/day)
Barbiturates			
amobarbital*	Amytal	Tablet: 15, 30, 50, 100 mg Capsule: 65, 200 mg Concentrate: 44 mg/5 ml (16-oz bottle) Parenteral: 250-, 500-mg vial	60–150
butabarbital*	Buticaps Butisol	Capsule: 15, 30 mg Tablet: 15, 30, 100, 150 mg Concentrate: 30 mg/5 ml (16-oz bottle)	100 45–120
mephobarbital*	Mebaral	Tablet: 32, 50, 100, 200 mg	150–200
pentobarbital*	Nembutal	Capsule: 30, 50, 100 mg Concentrate: 20 mg/ml (16-oz bottle) Parenteral: 50 mg/ml (2-ml ampule; 20-, 50-ml vial)	90–120 150–200 once (up to 500)
phenobarbital*	Multiple	Tablet and Capsule: multiple strengths Concentrate: 16 mg/ml; drops, 20 mg/5 ml elixir Parenteral: multiple-strength syringes, ampules, and vials	30–120

Carbamates			
meprobamate*	Equanil	Tablet: 200, 400 mg	1200–1600
	Miltown	Tablet: 200, 400, 600 mg	
Noradrenergic agents			
clonidine*	Catapres	Tablet: 0.1, 0.2, 0.3 mg	0.2–0.6
		Parenteral: 1 mg/ml (1-ml ampule)	
propranolol*	Inderal	Tablet: 10, 20, 40, 60, 80, 90 mg	60–160
Antihistamines			
hydroxyzine HCl*	Atarax	Tablet: 10, 25, 50, 100 mg	200–400
		Concentrate: 10 mg/5 ml (16-oz bottle)	
hydroxyzine pamoate*	Vistaril	Tablet: 25, 50, 100 mg	200–400
		Concentrate: 25 mg/5 ml	
		Parenteral: multiple-strength syringes and vials	50–100

Note. For information regarding antidepressants as anxiolytics, see Chapter 3.
* Available in generic form.

patient's subsequent behavior. Although in the past, amobarbital was administered intramuscularly several times a
day through prolonged psychotic excitements, there is no
real reason to believe that it is in fact regularly antipsychotic
or has any prolonged benefit. There is some suggestion that
too frequent use could result in either tolerance or, occasionally, delirium. Local experience in Boston suggests that
lorazepam, given intramuscularly in 1- to 2-mg doses, is as
useful as, and is safer than, amobarbital.

Intravenous amobarbital has been used in extreme emergency conditions in psychiatry to produce anesthetic-type
sleep within a few minutes. A dose of 150–200 mg given
over a period of 3–5 minutes intravenously could be used,
and additional doses up to 500 mg could be given if 250 mg
is not adequate to produce quiet sleep. If such "anesthetic"
use of amobarbital is being prescribed, the physician should
carefully watch the patient's breathing and vital signs and
give the medication slowly to make sure that respiration is
not suppressed. The major danger in addition to suppression
of the respiratory center in such treatment is the occasional
production of laryngospasm in patients with irritation of the
larynx and upper respiratory system. Barbiturates can of
course also produce crises in patients with acute intermittent
porphyria.

Intravenous amobarbital in doses of 100–300 mg, sometimes higher, has been used also in psychiatric conditions to
conduct Amytal interviews. When the amobarbital is injected
slowly over 5–10 minutes in most psychiatric patients, a
state of relaxation and mild intoxication with slurred speech
can be achieved during which patients will often talk more
easily and more volubly about their problems and past
experiences. Sometimes patients under these conditions will
reveal material not previously told to the psychiatrist. Although amobarbital has been called "truth serum," it is by
no means certain that stories told by patients under the

influence of amobarbital are likely to be any more truthful than stories told in the fully conscious state.

The Amytal interview was developed during World War II by Grinker and Spiegel (1945) as a treatment for severe combat fatigue. In the typical situation, soldiers emerged from combat essentially mute, shaking, paralyzed with fear, and looking blocked, dysphoric, and peculiar. They were either mute or unable to answer questions in more than monosyllables and appeared unable to cope emotionally with the traumatic events they had recently experienced. Under the influence of intravenous amobarbital, such soldiers often were able to give vivid and emotionally charged accounts of their horrifying experiences, and this form of catharsis often discharged their inner tensions and enabled them to function thereafter in a more normal and organized fashion with a substantially reduced level of anxiety. It is reasonable to believe that amobarbital might be of use in similar conditions that resemble some kind of acute traumatic stress syndrome encountered in clinical practice. Amytal interviews have also been used, often with some success, in patients with hysterical amnesia. Such patients can often, but by no means always, retrieve repressed memories for past events and give reasonable accounts of relevant portions of their past history. The interview can be used both in patients with isolated episodes of amnesia, for example for episodes of rape or assault or murder, or for patients who profess total amnesia for their entire past lives. Amobarbital given intravenously also is occasionally effective in resolving hysterical paralyses and other conversion symptoms.

Intravenous amobarbital also has a remarkable property in many patients in psychotic stupor. Although the stupor used to be generally referred to as catatonic stupor, there is currently some doubt whether individual cases of psychic mutism with frozen motor behavior are in fact a manifestation of schizophrenia or a manifestation of psychotic depression.

In either case, intravenous amobarbital given as in an Amytal interview can often produce a remarkable change in a patient's behavior. The frozen stupor will often clear remarkably, and the patient will be able to talk spontaneously, walk about, drink fluids, eat a meal, and otherwise carry on apparently normal activity for a half hour or sometimes for 2–3 hours. In some patients the psychotic material suppressed by the stupor becomes blatantly obvious as the patient talks about the delusions, hallucinations, and bizarre preoccupations. In other cases, the patient appears really quite normal without unusual thought content. Such patients often have no idea of why their behavior has become frozen and immobilized and why they are unable to speak or move. Obviously, the Amytal interview can occasionally be useful in the rare cases where a mute catatonic patient has been admitted to an emergency room or a psychiatric unit with no history and no identification and the clinician is unable to deduce even what the patient's name and address are, much less what the past history or probable psychiatric diagnosis is. In such situations, amobarbital given intravenously can be quite helpful in clarifying the situation. However, it should only be administered after all reasonable medical or pharmacological causes for such a mute or unresponsive state have been ruled out. Lorazepam, given intramuscularly, may be as useful as amobarbital sodium in relieving stupor.

MEPROBAMATE

Meprobamate occupies an intermediate position between the benzodiazepines and the barbiturates, both pharmacologically and historically. It was first marketed about 1956, having evolved from a chemically related muscle relaxant named mephenesin. Its structure is shown in Figure 6-3. Meprobamate has muscle relaxant and sedative properties, but it was initially evaluated as an antianxiety agent. On the basis of a small number of enthusiastic but uncontrolled

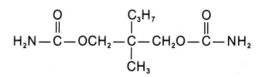

Figure 6-3. Chemical structure of meprobamate.

studies on anxiety, it was released to the market in the days when the FDA required only evidence of safety rather than evidence of efficacy. It became an instant national success with widespread publicity in the lay media.

Now that the dust has settled, some 30 years later, it is clear that meprobamate is, in fact, an effective antianxiety agent in the same sense that diazepam or chlordiazepoxide is effective, although controlled studies directly comparing the efficacy of meprobamate with benzodiazepines are almost nonexistent. The clinical dose of meprobamate is on the order of 400 mg three or four times a day, being approximately equivalent to 5 mg of diazepam three or four times a day (Table 6-3). The major side effects are sedation and malcoordination. The drug is relatively safe in overdose, less lethal than intermediate-acting barbiturates like pentobarbital, but a good deal less safe than diazepam. The drug produces physical dependence and tolerance in much the same way as do the barbiturates and the benzodiazepines. Significant withdrawal effects such as convulsions, agitation, or delirium occur after clinically relatively lower doses of meprobamate, for example, after 3,200 mg or eight 400-mg pills a day.

Currently, it is hard to identify any unique advantages possessed by meprobamate as an antianxiety drug. Among possible considerations, one should include the fact that it has been widely manufactured generically and therefore may be an inexpensive alternative to a patented benzodiazepine such as alprazolam or lorazepam. It is a reasonably effective and satisfactory hypnotic at a dose of 400–800 mg a day at bedtime. Clinically, we have seen occasional anxious patients who have a marked subjective intolerance to benzodiazepines becoming agitated, dysphoric, and restless on any of several of them. Some of these patients tolerate meprobamate quite well. It can also be used in those rare patients for whom an antianxiety drug is to be prescribed during the daytime, either as a prn medication or for 4–6 weeks. To our knowledge no one has evaluated meprobamate in such conditions as akathisia or panic disorder, where some benzodiazepines appear effective.

Deprol, a 35-year-old meprobamate-containing combination medication, deserves mention here. This combination of benactyzine and meprobamate is still marketed for use in depression. Each tablet contains 400 mg of meprobamate and 1 mg of benactyzine hydrochloride. There is essentially no evidence that benactyzine by itself is an effective antidepressant, although the compound is anticholinergic and might conceivably have some antidepressant properties. One trial in schizophrenic patients made many years ago shows benactyzine to increase hallucinatory and psychotic behavior. However, there are a handful of studies suggesting that Deprol is effective in some depressions and perhaps more effective than either of its ingredients. The question remains moot, and we have not heard of the compound being used clinically for a number of years. One of us recently prescribed Deprol to a patient who reported that it cost $2 per pill at her local pharmacy.

NORADRENERGIC AGENTS

In recent years, a number of studies have pointed to the potential use of beta-blockers (e.g., propranolol) and primarily presynaptic but also postsynaptic alpha$_2$-receptor agonists (e.g., clonidine) to ameliorate symptoms of anxiety. Use of these agents stems from the observations that certain symptoms (e.g., palpitations, sweating) of anxiety suggest involvement of the sympathetic nervous system. Investigations were first directed toward the use of beta-blockers in anxious musical performers. A number of years later, clonidine was shown by Gold et al. (1978) to be effective in blocking physiologic symptoms associated with opioid withdrawal, resulting in its eventual application to patients with anxiety disorders and possibly in nicotine withdrawal. This drug exerts alpha$_2$- (presynaptic) receptor agonist effects; however, since it is also a postsynaptic alpha$_2$ agonist, its pharmacologic actions are complex.

Clinical Indications, Names, and Structures

Beta-blockers (e.g., propranolol) are indicated for hypertension and for prophylaxis against angina, arrhythmias, migraine headaches, and hypertrophic subaortic stenosis. They are often quite useful in relieving akathisia in patients on neuroleptics, although they are not FDA approved for this use (see Chapter 4). They are also not FDA approved for use in anxiety, although several studies suggest propranolol may be useful. These studies were originally conducted in Great Britain and point to beta-blockers having particularly potent effects on the somatic manifestations of anxiety (e.g., palpitations, tremors) with less dramatic effects noted on the psychic component of anxiety. The antitremor properties of these drugs have resulted in their being commonly used in patients in whom hand tremors have developed secondary to lithium carbonate (see Chapter 5). A number of reports have suggested that although beta-blockers have some use in generalized anxiety, they are not particularly effective in blocking panic attacks. Indeed, Gorman et al. (1983) reported that propranolol failed to block lactate-induced panic attacks. However, some investigators have noted that propranolol may block panic anxiety resulting from isoproterenol (an adrenergic agonist) infusions and thus could still be effective in some patients with panic attacks.

Clonidine has an FDA indication for the treatment of hypertension. As noted above, it has been widely studied and used for blocking physiologic symptoms of opioid withdrawal (e.g., palpitations, sweating). The drug has also been studied in anxiety and in panic disorder and has been shown to be effective in both, although tolerance frequently develops to the antianxiety effects. It is conceivable that the drug's mixed, partial pre- and postsynaptic receptor agonist properties may enter into the development of tolerance. Clonidine has also been used to test various aspects of the catecholamine hypotheses of affective and anxiety disorders. Studies on nicotine withdrawal have yielded mixed results (see Chapter 11; Franks et al. 1989; Glassman et al. 1988). Generic and trade names of key noradrenergic agents are summarized in Table 6-3.

Dosage Ranges

Using propranolol as a model, clinicians should begin patients with peripheral symptoms of anxiety or with lithium-induced tremor at 10 mg bid and increase incrementally to approximately 60–160 mg/day (see Table 6-3). Although the usual maintenance dosage of the drug in patients with hypertension is as high as 240 mg/day, such dosages are rarely needed for anxious or tremulous patients. Generally, the use of these agents in patients with anxiety disorders should parallel that of the benzodiazepines, with attempts made at trying patients off the drug after a few weeks of treatment. In tremors secondary to lithium carbonate, many patients show a re-emergence of their tremors after discontinuation of the beta-blocker, resulting in their remaining on beta-blockers for prolonged periods. We know of no major untoward effects that have resulted; however, since some patients may become lethargic and even depressed on beta-blockers, clinicians need to keep this in mind in patients with a major affective disorder (see below). This is a confusing area since we have also used propranolol for tricyclic-induced tremor without affecting the depression in the vast majority of patients.

Clonidine should be started at a dose of 0.1 mg bid and increased by 0.1 mg every 1–2 days to a total daily dose of 0.4–0.6 mg (Table 6-3). Since some studies have indicated that tolerance develops to this drug, clinicians should attempt to limit the duration of exposure whenever possible.

Side Effects

Side effects of the beta-blockers include bradycardia, hypotension, weakness, fatigue, clouded sensorium, impotence, gastrointestinal upset, and bronchospasm, among others. For the psychiatrist, a few caveats appear warranted. Clinicians need to remember that these drugs are contraindicated in asthmatics because they may produce bronchospasm and in patients with Reynaud's disease because of the risk of increased peripheral vasoconstriction. Pindolol (Visken), which acts as a mixed beta-receptor agonist and antagonist, has less effect on receptors that control bronchial constriction and has been argued to be potentially safe in patients with asthma. However, its marked agonist effects can result in unpleasant stimulation, and we have not found it particularly useful in anxious patients. As for the capacity of beta-blockers to cause depression, we have not seen patients who have developed true depressive disorders. Rather, we have noted that some patients may feel "washed out" or lethargic. However, clinicians at other institutions have reported cases of propranolol-induced depression with endogenous features that remit with discontinuation of the drug. One strategy is to switch to a beta-blocker, such as atenolol, that is less lipophilic and that exerts less central nervous system effects. This strategy may be particularly useful in men who have experienced decreased sexual potency on propranolol. When stopping beta-blockers, it is wisest to taper the dose to avoid any rebound phenomena that could result in untoward cardiac or blood pressure effects.

Clonidine also has a relatively favorable side-effect profile. Its major side effects include dry mouth, sedation or fatigue, and hypotension. In hypertensive patients, bid scheduling (with two-thirds of the dose given at the hour of sleep) has been advocated to deal with its sedating effects. Discontinuation should be gradual to avoid rebound or the hypertensive crises that have been reported in hypertensive patients who were suddenly withdrawn from the drug.

ANTIDEPRESSANTS AS ANXIOLYTIC AGENTS

Agoraphobia and Panic

Several antidepressants exert major antianxiety effects. Imipramine was first reported by Klein and colleagues in the 1960s to have potent anxiolytic effects in agoraphobic patients with panic. Clinically, it appears that most, if not all, TCAs exert similar antipanic effects. In addition, the monoamine oxidase inhibitor (MAOI) phenelzine is also a potent antipanic agent, as the other MAOIs and trazodone probably are. However, not all antidepressants are as effective in panic. Most notably, bupropion appears not to exert antipanic effects as reliably. The noradrenergic effects of various antidepressants (particularly the TCAs and MAOIs) on the locus coeruleus generally have been invoked to explain their antipanic activity. Whether this explains the possible antipanic effects of trazodone is unclear. In addition, fluoxetine appears to block panic attacks in some patients. Bupropion exerts virtually no effect on noradrenergic systems.

Early on, the general rule of thumb was that panic patients required only low doses of TCAs (e.g., 50 mg/day of imipramine) to respond. In the past few years, it has become more evident that, as in depression, many panic patients require relatively higher doses of TCAs or MAOIs, although a small proportion are very sensitive to TCAs, tolerating only 10–25 mg of imipramine a day. We recommend using the general dosage regimens of TCAs in depression (see Chapter 3).

It appears that panic patients may be quite sensitive to the stimulatory properties of fluoxetine and require extremely low doses (e.g., 5–10 mg/day, dissolved in juice or water) at initiation of treatment.

Generalized Anxiety Disorder

Recently, collaborative studies have pointed out that TCAs also exert effects in generalized anxiety disorder. In one major study, imipramine was as effective at 4–6 weeks as the benzodiazepine chlordiazepoxide in patients with this disorder. However, in the first 2 weeks, the benzodiazepine was more effective. Given the need for rapid improvement and the greater side effects with TCAs, the TCAs should not be viewed as first-line drugs in generalized anxiety disorder. They can be used in patients who do not respond quickly to benzodiazepines.

Social Phobia

Seriously symptomatic patients with social phobia suffer marked anxiety in one or more "social" situations—eating in public, signing checks, public speaking, or even being in large groups. The condition, as defined in DSM-III-R, may include more limited fears of performing or speaking in public, often called *performance anxiety*. Performance anxiety is less incapacitating than other social phobias but may affect, of course, an area vital to a patient's career.

There is reasonable evidence that milder degrees of performance anxiety studied in volunteers (e.g., music students) respond to beta-blockers given a couple of hours before the performance. Several beta-blockers, including propranolol, oxprenolol, pindolol, and atenolol, have been more effective than placebo in individual controlled studies. Atenolol is cardioselective and may not cross the blood-brain barrier well, suggesting that beta-blockers may act, at least in part, by suppressing tachycardia and tremor.

For more symptomatic social phobias, MAOIs appear to be the treatment of choice. The only study solely involving social phobias by Liebowitz et al. (1986), though open, was strongly positive. Most of their patients had significantly less symptom relief on a beta-blocker. Several other studies of MAOIs in mixed groups of agoraphobic and social phobic patients were not separated out for analysis. In studies comparing amitriptyline and phenelzine, the MAOI was superior to the tricyclic on rating scale measures of social discomfort, suggesting that tricyclics in general may be less effective in social phobia.

Clomipramine has been studied in mixed groups of phobic patients with good effect. Social phobic patients were included in the samples but their responses were not reported separately, and modern diagnostic criteria were not used.

On the basis of limited evidence, mild social and/or performance anxiety could be treated first with a beta-blocker, and more impaired patients could be given phenelzine. Clomipramine could be tried in patients adverse to trying MAOIs or in patients who failed on MAOIs previously, either because of side effects or lack of improvement.

Posttraumatic Stress Disorder

Posttraumatic stress disorder (PTSD) is included among the anxiety disorders in DSM-III-R. The condition, as manifested in combat veterans, has been recognized for many years. More recently, however, patients who have experienced sexual or physical abuse in childhood are presenting with similar clusters of symptoms. PTSD patients usually show moderate degrees of anxiety and depression, "intrusive" symptoms such as nightmares and flashbacks, and intrusive recollections of traumatic events plus "avoidance" symptoms such as emotional numbing, distance from loved ones, and active suppression of memories of bad events. Dissociative episodes also occur.

Explanatory pathophysiologic mechanisms include chronic, high levels of sympathetic nervous system activity and kindling, a process by which small recurring stimuli to the brain lead gradually to progressively larger overreactions and ultimately to seizures. Sleep patterns in PTSD in veterans are dissimilar to those found in depression. PTSD patients show increased, not decreased, rapid eye movement (REM) latency, reduced total REM sleep, and reduced stage 4 sleep.

Research on response to drug therapies in PTSD is limited in scope and quality. Open studies have suggested that both TCAs and MAOIs are useful in some patients at conventional dosages. The one published controlled study by Frank et al. (1988) shows both imipramine and phenelzine to be more effective than placebo; however, they provide only partial symptomatic relief. Because many patients with PTSD may also have major substance abuse problems, TCAs may be safer. MAOIs may help PTSD patients with clear panic attacks. Fluoxetine has not been studied under double-blind conditions; however, a local expert believes it is the best of the antidepressants for this condition.

Open studies also suggest that autonomic drugs such as clonidine and propranolol help reduce symptoms of PTSD. Lithium may reduce overreactions to minor stresses and feelings of being out of control. Carbamazepine may have a similar effect. Antipsychotics are thought to be helpful.

Benzodiazepines as hypnotics can help with sleep disturbance but carry with them the potential for abuse. There is a general clinical belief that ongoing group or individual psychotherapy should accompany drug therapy. None of the drug therapies listed above are regularly and completely effective in PTSD, and some treatment-resistant PTSD patients end up on complex and ineffective multiple medication regimens without obvious improvement. These patients present a challenge to pharmacotherapists and psychotherapists alike.

Obsessive-Compulsive Disorder

A small number of case reports in the literature describe favorable responses in obsessive-compulsive patients being treated with almost any available medications, including antipsychotic drugs, lithium, TCAs, and MAOIs. All of these probably work in occasional patients, although one would guess that antipsychotic drugs are more helpful in schizophrenic patients with marked obsessive-compulsive features, and drugs commonly used in depression are most effective in alleviating secondary depression when it is superimposed on the obsessive-compulsive disorder itself.

However, there is a large battery of clinical lore from Europe and from individual practitioners in the United States that asserts that clomipramine (Anafranil) is substantially better than most other drug therapies in obsessive-compulsive disorder. Insel et al. (1983) at the National Institute of Mental Health (NIMH) carried out consecutive open studies of clomipramine, desipramine, and zimelidine and reported clomipramine to be most effective, zimelidine somewhat effective, and desipramine ineffective. Results of a large double-blind study comparing clomipramine with placebo in obsessive-compulsive disorder in the United States were recently reported. The results show that clomipramine is strikingly more effective than placebo. About 50% of the drug-treated patients showed improvement in comparison to 1–2% on placebo. This finding conforms to Insel's experience and the clinical impressions of many psychopharmacologists. Clomipramine is believed to cause gradual and progressive improvement in obsessive-compulsive symptoms, more impressive in the second month of treatment than in the first.

Clomipramine is a potent serotonin reuptake blocker, and this action has been proposed to underlie the anti-obsessive-compulsive effect. However, the drug is demethylated in humans, and the resultant metabolite is a potent norepinephrine reuptake blocker.

It is difficult to make a firm recommendation about the drug of choice in the treatment of obsessive-compulsive disorder. Clomipramine, which was released in February 1990, certainly has the best evidence for efficacy but only elicits major improvement in about half the cases treated. It has a variety of side effects. Most are those to be expected of a TCA with a profile similar to imipramine—dry mouth, constipation, hypotension, tachycardia—but, based on the literature on its use in depression, clomipramine appears to cause a somewhat higher incidence of sweating, tremor, and anorgasmia than other tricyclics and may be more likely to cause seizures at higher dosages. Fluoxetine, which has been less well studied in obsessive-compulsive disorder, may be better tolerated. It is unclear whether it is as effective, but some open studies have been positive. Fluvoxamine has been studied under double-blind conditions. It appears effective in this condition; however, it produces high rates of nausea and may be less effective than clomipramine.

It is worth noting that clomipramine is widely held to be a very effective antidepressant in Europe. However, the published evidence, which mainly consists of open trials and small trials comparing clomipramine with other antidepressants, is weak. The drug comes out as about equal to older antidepressants in efficacy. It probably is effective in panic-agoraphobia as well.

The dosage of clomipramine is similar to that of imipramine or amitriptyline—a starting dose of 25 mg/day gradually increased to 150 mg/day as tolerated, going higher if no clinical improvement is noted after 3 or 4 weeks. The maximum daily dosage is 250 mg/day because above that seizures have been reported to be more common. Blood levels for clomipramine and desmethylclomipramine should be obtainable from standard clinical laboratories, but relationships between improvement in either obsessive-compulsive disorder or depression and blood levels are not at all clear at this point.

ANTIHISTAMINES

The antihistamine hydroxyzine enjoys indications for the treatment of anxiety and tension associated with psychoneurotic conditions or physical disease states. It is also indicated in the treatment of pruritis due to allergic conditions and for pre- and postoperative sedation. In psychiatric practice, antihistamines are less commonly used in treating anxious patients, reflecting their less potent anxiolytic effects.

Hydroxyzine's recommended oral dosage in adults is 50–100 mg qid (Table 6-3). The major side effects include drowsiness and dry mouth. It does not produce physical dependence. It may produce central nervous system depression when added to alcohol, narcotic analgesics, central nervous system depressants, and TCAs. The antihistamine diphenhydramine is commonly used in medicine and psychiatry as a sedative-hypnotic (see Chapter 7).

BUSPIRONE

The development of buspirone—a nonbenzodiazepine, generally nonsedating anxiolytic—stirred considerable excitement in psychopharmacologic circles. It represented the first prominent anxiolytic to be introduced since the benzodiazepines. The drug was originally developed as a potential antipsychotic agent. However, it was found in early clinical trials to have little antipsychotic potency but was eventually

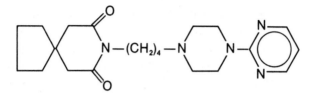

Figure 6-4. Chemical structure of buspirone.

shown to have antiaggression effects in primates and antianxiety effects in humans. Buspirone is marketed under the brand name of Buspar. Its structure is shown in Figure 6-4.

The drug does not bind with high affinity to benzodiazepine and GABA receptors, although it may have an effect on the chloride channel coupled to the benzodiazepine-GABA complex. Buspirone has little antiseizure effect. Its anxiolytic effects were originally postulated to be via dopaminergic properties, although the drug's central dopaminergic effects are not entirely clear. Some investigators had argued that buspirone exerted potent presynaptic dopamine antagonist effects resulting in increased dopamine at the synapses. Others noted that the drug also had peripheral postsynaptic dopamine blocking properties. More recently, buspirone has also been reported to exert effects on serotonin-1A receptors to decrease firing of neurons in the raphe.

The apparent advantages of buspirone lie in its not being sedating at the usual anxiolytic dosages and having little potential for addiction or abuse. Wider clinical use has not shown the drug to have major untoward effects. Although buspirone was found to be as effective as traditional benzodiazepines under double-blind conditions in the treatment of patients with generalized anxiety disorder, many practitioners have found the drug to be a disappointment in terms of overall efficacy. There are a number of possible explanations: inadequate dosing and/or low potency of the drug; lack of sedative properties causing a necessary, but difficult, waiting period for anxiolysis; and previous benzodiazepine exposure. Schweizer and colleagues (1986) reported poorer response in patients who had previously been exposed to benzodiazepines, suggesting that previous, more immediate responses to benzodiazepines may lead to disappointment with a slower or more gradually acting agent. The drug has not been shown to be effective in panic. There are preliminary data to suggest that the drug may have potential benefit in anxious patients with chronic obstructive pulmonary disease. Also, recent data suggest that the drug may have antidepressant properties at doses of 30–60 mg/day and that it can be used to augment the antiobsessive effects of clomipramine or fluoxetine.

The dosage of buspirone is similar to that of diazepam. The average daily dosage is 15–25 mg/day with an initial dose of 5 mg bid. At single doses of 20–40 mg, the drug produces sedation or dysphoria. At one time, the general recommendation for switching patients from benzodiazepines to buspirone was to taper the benzodiazepine before starting buspirone. The rationale was that buspirone would not block benzodiazepine withdrawal. However, this was difficult for patients to tolerate and probably led to poor acceptance of the drug in some patients. It seems more reasonable to add buspirone to the benzodiazepine regimen and to stabilize the buspirone dosage first. Thereafter, the benzodiazepine dosage can be tapered.

Side effects include headache, nausea, dizziness, and tension, which generally are not major problems. Indeed, the drug appears to have a more desirable side-effect profile than do the benzodiazepines. It does not appear to impair motor coordination and shows little untoward interaction with alcohol. According to an old report, the drug may exacerbate psychosis in schizoaffective patients, reflecting complex pro-dopaminergic properties. This has not been a problem in clinical usage in the United States.

Bibliography

Ballenger JC, Burrows GD, DuPont RL Jr, et al: Alprazolam in panic disorder and agoraphobia: results from a multicenter trial, I: efficacy in short-term treatment. Arch Gen Psychiatry 45:413–422, 1988

Baxter LR, Thompson JM, Schwartz JM, et al: Trazodone treatment response in obsessive-compulsive disorders correlated with shifts in glucose metabolism in the caudate nuclei. Psychopathology 20(5):114–122, 1987

Benzodiazepine seizures: an update. International Drug Therapy Newsletter 24:5–7, 1989

Braestrup C, Squires RF: Brain specific benzodiazepine receptors. Br J Psychiatry 133:249–260, 1978

DeVeaugh-Geiss J, Landau P, Katz R: Preliminary results from a multicenter trial of clomipramine in obsessive-compulsive disorder. Psychopharmacol Bull 25:36–40, 1989

Frank JB, Kosten TR, Giller EL, et al: A randomized clinical trial of phenelzine and imipramine for PTSD. Am J Psychiatry 145:1289–1291, 1988

Friedman MJ: Toward a rational pharmacotherapy for PTSD: an interim report. Am J Psychiatry 145:281–285, 1988

Fyer AJ, Liebowitz MR, Gorman JM, et al: Discontinuation of alprazolam treatment in panic patients. Am J Psychiatry 144:303–308, 1987

Gold MS, Redmond DE Jr, Kleber HD: Clonidine in opiate withdrawal. Lancet 1:929–930, 1978

Goldberg HL: Buspirone hydrochloride: a unique new anxiolytic agent: pharmacokinetics, clinical pharmacology, abuse potential and clinical efficacy. Pharmacotherapy 4:315–324, 1984

Gorman JM, Levy GF, Liebowitz MR, et al: Effect of acute beta-adrenergic blockade or lactate induced panic. Arch Gen Psychiatry 40:1079–1082, 1983

Granville-Grossman KL, Turner P: The effect of propranolol on anxiety. Lancet 1:788–790, 1966

Greenblatt DJ, Shader RI, Abernethy DR: Current status of benzodiazepines [first of two parts]. N Engl J Med 309:354–359, 1983

Greenblatt DJ, Shader RI, Abernethy DR: Current status of benzodiazepines [second of two parts]. N Engl J Med 309:410–415, 1983

Grinker R, Spiegel J: Men under stress. Philadelphia, PA, Blakiston, 1945

Herman JB, Rosenbaum JF, Brotman AW: The alprazolam to clonazepam switch for the treatment of panic disorder. J Clin Psychopharmacol 7:175–178, 1987

Insel TR (ed): New Findings in Obsessive-Compulsive Disorder. Washington, DC, American Psychiatric Press, 1984

Insel TR, Murphy DL, Cohen RM, et al: Obsessive compulsive disorder: a double-blind trial of clomipramine and clorgyline. Arch Gen Psychiatry 40:605–612, 1983

Isbell H, Altschul S, Kornetsky C, et al: Chronic barbiturate intoxication: an experimental study. AMA Archives of Neurology and Psychiatry 64:1–28, 1950

Kahn R, McNair D, Covi L, et al: Effects of psychotropic agents in high anxiety subjects. Psychopharmacol Bull 17:97–100, 1981

Klein DF: Importance of psychiatric diagnosis in prediction of clinical drug effects. Arch Gen Psychiatry 16:118–126, 1967

Klein E, Uhde TW, Post RM: Preliminary evidence for the utility of carbamazepine in alprazolam withdrawal. Am J Psychiatry 143:235–236, 1986

Lader M: Summary and commentary, in Pharmacology of Benzodiazepines. Edited by Usdin E, Skolnick P, Tallman JF, et al. New York, Macmillan, 1982, pp 53–60

Liebowitz MR, Fyer AJ, McGrath P, et al: Clonidine treatment of panic disorder. Psychopharmacol Bull 17:122–123, 1981

Liebowitz MR, Gorman JM, Fyer AJ, et al: Social phobia: review of a neglected anxiety disorder. Arch Gen Psychiatry 42:729–736, 1985

Liebowitz MR, Fyer AJ, Gorman JM, et al: Phenelzine in social phobia. J Clin Psychopharmacol 6:93–98, 1986

Lucki I, Rickels K, Geller AM: Chronic use of benzodiazepines and psychomotor and cognitive test performance. Psychopharmacology 88:426–433, 1986

Meltzer HY, Fleming R, Robertson A: The effect of buspirone on prolactin and growth hormone secretion in man. Arch Gen Psychiatry 40:1099–1102, 1983

Menza M, Harris D: Benzodiazepines and catatonia: an overview. Biol Psychiatry 26:842–846, 1989

Mooney JJ, Schatzberg AF, Cole JO, et al: Enhanced signal transduction by adenylate cyclase in platelet membranes of patients showing antidepressant responses to alprazolam: preliminary data. J Psychiatr Res 19:65–75, 1985

Noyes R, Anderson DJ, Clancy J, et al: Diazepam and propranolol in panic disorder and agoraphobia. Arch Gen Psychiatry 41:287–292, 1984

Noyes R Jr, DuPont RL Jr, Pecknold JC, et al: Alprazolam in panic disorder and agoraphobia: results from a multicenter trial, II: patient acceptance, side effects, and safety. Arch Gen Psychiatry 45:423–428, 1988

Pecknold JC, Swinson RP, Kuch K, et al: Alprazolam in panic disorder and agoraphobia: results from a multicenter trial, III: discontinuation effects. Arch Gen Psychiatry 45:429–436, 1988

Pollack MH, Tesar GE, Rosenbaum JF, et al: Clonazepam in the treatment of panic disorder and agoraphobias: a one-year follow-up. J Clin Psychopharmacol 6:302–304, 1986

Problems associated with alprazolam therapy. International Drug Therapy Newsletter 23:29–31, 1988

Rickels K, Chase WG, Downing RW: Long-term diazepam therapy and clinical outcome. JAMA 250:767–771, 1983

Rickels K, Schweizer E, Csanalosi I, et al: Long-term treatment of anxiety and risk of withdrawal: prospective comparison of clorazepate and buspirone. Arch Gen Psychiatry 45:444–450, 1988

Ries RK, Roy-Byrne PP, Ward NG, et al: Carbamazepine treatment for benzodiazepine withdrawal. Am J Psychiatry 146:536–537, 1989

Sathanathan GL, Sanzhavi F, Phillips N: MJ 9022 (buspirone): correlation between neuroleptic potential and stereotypy. Current Therapeutic Research 18:701–705, 1975

Schweizer E, Rickels K, Lucki I: Resistance to the antianxiety effect of buspirone in patients with a history of benzodiazepine use (letter). N Engl J Med 314:719–720, 1986

Sethy VH: Pharmacokinetic studies of triazolobenzodiazepines by drug-receptor binding assays, in Pharmacology of Benzodiazepines. Edited by Usdin E, Skolnick P, Tallman JF, et al. New York, Macmillan, 1982

Sheehan DV, Ballenger J, Jacobsen G: Treatment of endogenous anxiety with phobic, hysterical, and hypochondriacal symptoms. Arch Gen Psychiatry 37:51–59, 1980

Swedo SE, Leonard HL, Rapoport JL, et al: A double-blind comparison of clomipramine and desipramine in the treatment of trichotillomania (hair pulling). N Engl J Med 321:497–501, 1989

Tesar GE, Rosenbaum JF: Successful use of clonazepam in patients with treatment-resistant panic disorder. J Nerv Ment Dis 174:447–482, 1986

Tyrer PJ, Lader MH: Clinical response to propranolol and diazepam in somatic and psychic anxiety. Br Med J 2:14–16, 1974

Tyrer P, Shawcross C: Monoamine oxidase inhibitors in anxiety disorders. J Psychiatr Res 22 (suppl 1):87–98, 1988

van der Kolk BA: The drug treatment of post-traumatic stress disorder. J Affective Disord 13:203–213, 1987

Zitrin CM, Klein DF, Woerner MG: Treatment of phobias, I: comparison of imipramine hydrochloride and placebo. Arch Gen Psychiatry 40:125–138, 1983

Hypnotics

7

Insomnia is a common problem that is troubling enough for many patients to seek help from psychiatrists or sleep disorder specialists. Many patients complain, often despairingly, of very poor sleep or total insomnia, but nevertheless appear on all-night sleep recordings or nurses' or relatives' observations to be sleeping most of the night. Attempts to objectify insomnia in terms of the time it takes for the person to fall asleep or the length of time actually slept have often not proved useful. Also, the psychiatrist is not uncommonly faced with patients who are actually awake all night, particularly those with marked depression and anxiety, whose sleep is so disturbed that they feel exhausted the next day and claim that they "can't function."

In psychiatric patients, troublesome insomnia is often one feature of a wider symptom complex, which may also include diurnal rhythm disturbances of activity, mood, etc. Depressed patients classically have early morning awakening and diurnal variation. Some, however, have marked difficulty falling asleep as well. Patients with pronounced initial insomnia may be separated into those who sleep fitfully and poorly even after falling asleep and those who do sleep well after even several hours of initial insomnia. Such patients can sleep from 4:00 A.M. until noon. A few patients with very severe depression complain of almost complete insomnia, claiming they lie in bed all night without sleeping, often experiencing dysphoric, miserable ruminations.

Other psychiatric conditions are also manifested by sleep disturbances. Patients with anxiety disorders are more likely to have trouble falling asleep. Those with mania or hypomania may stay up all night either happily overactive or dysphorically agitated, as may patients with schizophrenia or schizophreniform psychoses. Classically, manic patients do not complain of sleeplessness but rather claim that they do not *need* to sleep. Demented organic patients may become more confused and agitated toward evening (sundowner syndrome) and may also be agitated at night after having slept all day. Patients very upset by major stress—e.g., bereavement, rejections, or physical trauma—may have insomnia as part of an acute stress response.

Insomnia in all of the relatively acute psychiatric conditions mentioned above is fairly straightforward to treat. Insomnia as part of a depressive disorder almost always responds to a standard antidepressant—in fact, some of the more sedative antidepressants (amitriptyline, doxepin, trimipramine, trazodone) may be useful hypnotics even in the absence of depression. For depression with poor sleep, it is sensible to begin with a sedative antidepressant (see Chapter 3), but even more stimulant antidepressants such as protriptyline, desipramine, or fluoxetine usually improve sleep as the depressive syndrome improves. In manic and schizophrenic excitements and in some organic agitations, the insomnia responds well to antipsychotic drugs of any class, although chlorpromazine and thioridazine may initially be slightly more effective as hypnotics before the general syndrome ameliorates.

Thus, the best general approach is to treat the psychiatric condition that underlies the insomnia with drugs that are appropriate to that condition rather than prescribing a benzodiazepine or other hypnotic drug first for the insomnia and then treating the depression or psychosis later.

In principle, a psychiatrist can run an inpatient ward or treat outpatients without ever prescribing a hypnotic. In practice, however, life often is (or appears to be) more complicated. Other patients, families, and nursing staff members become very upset if patients do not retire to bed and sleep without disturbing them. Often, hypnotics end up being prescribed to cut down on distress in the patient and his or her milieu. Such prescribing is often justifiable but can pose problems. First, the hypnotic may not put the patient to sleep but instead may leave the patient groggy, confused, and even more agitated. Second, a long-acting hypnotic, like flurazepam, may leave the patient groggy the next day. Third, once the patient is used to getting a hypnotic (and the doctor is used to prescribing it), the practice may continue for weeks or even months, long after the initial phase of the illness or the stress of hospitalization has passed. When the sleeping pill is finally stopped, rebound insomnia is likely to occur and lead to resumption of the hypnotic to control it. In fact, in the case of short-acting benzodiazepine hypnotics such as triazolam, rebound insomnia can even occur 4 hours after taking the medication. This can precipitate overutilization of the compound with some patients taking additional dosages to help them fall back asleep.

Another problem is the new patient being admitted to the hospital (or visiting a new psychiatrist) who is thoroughly accustomed to taking, for months or years, 60 mg of flurazepam or 2000 mg of chloral hydrate at bedtime but who still complains of poor sleep, which is, of course, reportedly much worse if the hypnotic is stopped. Here, the obvious options are to taper the hypnotic gradually while treating the major psychiatric disorder or to continue it while dealing with the core condition. The difficulty with the second, interpersonally easier option is that the hypnotic may never in fact be discontinued. A more complicated version of this scenario is the patient who comes to the psychiatrist while on several psychoactive drugs of different classes, all of which need to be withdrawn or changed. In this situation, it is common to leave the hypnotic at a stable dose and taper and stop the other drugs first to avoid confusing the effects of stopping the hypnotic with the already potentially complex effects of also discontinuing a tricyclic antidepressant (TCA) or an antipsychotic.

At present, the only real indications for hypnotics in insomnia are for brief (3- to 7-day) use or occasional use in transitory insomnia caused either by acute life stresses or by major shifts in diurnal rhythm, as in jet lag or changing from one work shift to another.

Although it is wise to avoid prolonged hypnotic usage, prolonged use of a benzodiazepine hypnotic may be less harmful than is often said and may in fact provide some benefit. The available evidence from sleep laboratories suggests that hypnotics improve sleep measurably for only about a week, but many confirmed hypnotic users swear that the hypnotics are *always* helpful and even vitally necessary. Perhaps the initial sedation at peak blood level provides a familiar conditioned cue conducive to falling asleep. Certainly, some patients who have taken hypnotics every night for several years continue to complain of poor sleep and daytime fatigue and dysphoria for months after the hypnotic has been stopped. A sleep expert can often prove helpful in the treatment of chronic insomnia with persistent hypnotic dependence by using behavioral techniques.

Some patients who present to psychiatrists may actually suffer from a primary sleep disorder or have a sleep disorder secondary to medications. In patients in whom insomnia is a major or primary complaint, sleep apnea should be considered as a diagnosis, especially if snoring with irregular respiration is noted by the patient's bedmate. Nocturnal myoclonus may result in extremely disturbed sleep characterized by thrashing about. The condition often responds to 1–3 mg of clonazepam at bedtime. Narcolepsy on occasion will present as atypical depression with fatigue and hypersomnia and can be treated with stimulants and perhaps protriptyline. On the other hand, excessive intake of stimulants—caffeine and diet pills, as well as phenylpropanolamine used in treatment of sinus disorders, cough, or asthma—may cause insomnia.

Insomnia, often quite troublesome, can also occur as a complication of psychotropic therapy. Some patients develop insomnia if stimulant tricyclics (desipramine and protriptyline) are given at bedtime, and a few patients even develop insomnia on all—or many—tricyclics, including amitriptyline. Our experience has been that doxepin or trimipramine is more likely to be tolerated by such patients. Sometimes moving the tricyclic from bedtime administration to daytime will resolve this problem. Fluoxetine and bupropion may also cause insomnia and thus are generally not given at bedtime. In our experience, early initial insomnia in fluoxetine-treated patients does not augur poor antidepressant response.

The monoamine oxidase inhibitors (MAOIs) can produce severe insomnia in patients showing an otherwise excellent response. Often this insomnia is not initially bothersome; however, some patients do become very troubled by a reduction of sleep of 4 or more hours. This is often accompanied by daytime fatigue and sleepiness. Shifting the dose to early in the day usually does not help. These patients may require hypnotics, trazodone, or low-dose amitriptyline or trimipramine (see Chapters 3 and 9).

HYPNOTIC BENZODIAZEPINES

The benzodiazepines are the most widely prescribed sedative-hypnotics in the United States today. Although most benzodiazepines have hypnotic properties, as of 1989 only three benzodiazepines enjoyed an indication as a hypnotic—flurazepam, temazepam, and triazolam.

The principles for discriminating among these three drugs are similar to those described in Chapter 6 for the anxiolytic benzodiazepines—structure, pharmacokinetics, absorption, and distribution (Table 7-1). For example, each of these hypnotics belongs to a separate structural subclass: 2-keto (flurazepam), 3-hydroxy (temazepam), and triazolo (triazolam) (Figure 7-1).

The metabolism and half-lives of these subclass members parallel their anxiolytic counterparts. Flurazepam is oxidized in the liver, and, like diazepam, it has a relatively long half-life (40 hours) and also forms a long-acting (100 hours) metabolite, desalkyflurazepam. Temazepam is conjugated with a glucuronide radical in the liver and has a much shorter half-life (8 hours) and no active metabolites. Triazolam is oxidized but with no clearly active metabolites and enjoys an extremely short half-life (3–6 hours) (Table 7-1).

The absorptions of flurazepam and triazolam are more rapid (peak blood levels occur at 30 and 20 minutes, respectively) than that of temazepam, which may not be absorbed for 45–60 minutes. The slower absorption accounts for patients not falling asleep rapidly after taking this medication. Clinicians should advise patients to take temazepam approximately 1 hour before retiring to avoid anticipatory discomfort and their resorting to premature repeat dosing.

A new benzodiazepine hypnotic, quazepam, has recently been released. Chemically, it does not fall into any of the three classes described in Chapter 6. However, the drug's pharmacokinetics place it in the same range as flurazepam because the drug and its metabolite have half-lives of about 40 hours. Metabolism and elimination are slowed in the elderly. This pattern suggests that sedation the next morning should be more of a problem than early rebound insomnia. Quazepam's only "special" feature is that it binds selectively

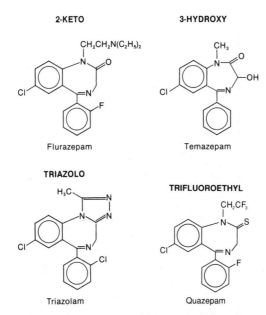

Figure 7-1. Chemical structures of hypnotic benzodiazepines.

to Type 1 benzodiazepine receptors, whereas flurazepam and other older benzodiazepines bind equally to both Type 1 and Type 2 sites in the brain. There is no evidence that this special binding property is of particular clinical value. Quazepam is a long-acting hypnotic, probably similar to flurazepam in its clinical utility. It is available in 7.5-mg and 15-mg tablets.

The distribution of the sedative benzodiazepines is relatively rapid. Indeed, the acute formation of high peak blood levels is thought to account for why patients fall asleep relatively quickly on these drugs. The decline from peak levels may account for why patients can awaken often, even when they still show significant drug plasma levels. Moreover, the decline from peak levels and the need for peak levels to induce sleep also explain why patients treated with longer-acting benzodiazepines like flurazepam require nightly dosages.

Some investigators and clinicians have argued that a non-

Table 7-1. Hypnotic benzodiazepines

Generic name	Brand name	Dosage form	Dosage (mg/day)	Absorption	Major active components	Approximate half-life (hours)
flurazepam*	Dalmane	Capsule: 15, 30 mg	15–30	Intermediate	hydroxyethyl-flurazepam desalkylflurazepam	1 100
quazepam	Doral	Capsule: 7.5, 15 mg	7.5–15	Intermediate	oxoquazepam desalkyl-oxoquazepam	39 73
temazepam*	Restoril	Capsule: 15, 30 mg	15–30	Intermediate to slow	temazepam	9
triazolam	Halcion	Tablet: 0.125, 0.25, 0.5 mg	0.125–0.5	Intermediate	triazolam	3

* Available in generic form.

long-acting compound (e.g., temazepam) offers great advantages because it is largely excreted before the next morning. Although at least one study has pointed to the safe use of triazolam for inducing sleep on transatlantic flights and preventing jet lag, as discussed above, there may be disadvantages associated with very short acting hypnotics—particularly rebound insomnia and anterograde amnesia. Rebound insomnia represents a worsening of sleep disturbance occurring soon after discontinuing the hypnotic. With the short-acting hypnotics, this occurs within the first two nights after discontinuation and can be troublesome for patients. Although acutely apparent with shorter-acting compounds, it may occur 5–7 days after discontinuation of benzodiazepines with longer half-lives and may be misinterpreted as a reemergence of the underlying insomnia rather than as a rebound phenomenon. When rebound insomnia occurs, clinicians should avoid resumption of the drug. Rather, reassurance and the prescription of antihistamine sedatives (e.g., 50 mg of diphenhydramine) or sedating antidepressants (e.g., 50–100 mg of trazodone) for a few days may prove beneficial. When this does not work, reinstituting the benzodiazepine and gradually tapering the dose is an alternative strategy.

The side effects of the sedative-hypnotic benzodiazepines are similar to those of their anxiolytic counterparts. They include sedation, ataxia, anterograde amnesia, slurred speech, and nausea. These side effects are not particularly dangerous, although sedation can be a problem if the individual attempts to drive, to operate heavy machinery, etc. There is weak evidence to suggest that the longer half-life compounds cause clinically important cognitive problems the following day; however, this area has not been well studied. Refined and detailed psychological testing can usually detect impairment of cognitive or psychomotor function the morning after a benzodiazepine hypnotic has been used to induce sleep. The real question is whether this impairment is clinically important; the vast majority of hypnotic users do not note behavioral impairment the next day unless they also note persistent sedation as well. However, as noted above, there are several reports of pronounced anterograde amnesia ("blackouts") in patients treated with triazolam. Indeed, some healthy individuals who have used triazolam to induce sleep during a transatlantic flight have described not remembering arriving in Europe or what they did the next day.

One possible problem with longer-acting benzodiazepines is illustrated by a patient treated with flurazepam nightly for years, who was shifted to an equivalent dose of temazepam. He developed a clear benzodiazepine withdrawal syndrome; the shorter-acting drug could not adequately replace the longer-acting one.

BARBITURATES

A number of barbiturates enjoy FDA indications for usage as sedative-hypnotics. These compounds are listed in Table 7-2. Pentobarbital, secobarbital, amobarbital, and a combination of secobarbital and amobarbital are most commonly used for nighttime sedation. In addition, several of these enjoy indications for both day and nighttime sedation. (The use of amobarbital, butisol, and other barbiturates for daytime sedation is discussed in Chapter 6.) Dosage ranges of these compounds and routes of administration are also listed in Table 7-2. Structures are shown in Figure 6-2.

For many years barbiturates were widely used for their hypnotic effects, but their use has dwindled with the introduction of the safer benzodiazepines. The half-lives of barbiturates determine their clinical applications. The extremely short-acting barbiturates (e.g., hexobarbital) are used for preanesthesia or anesthesia. Intermediate-duration barbiturates (e.g., pentobarbital) are used for induction and maintenance of sleep. Longer-acting compounds may be used for agitation or anxiety (see Chapter 6). Barbiturate preparations are variations of a barbituric acid structure with substitutions

Table 7-2. Barbiturates for insomnia

Generic name	Brand name	Dosage forms	Nighttime dosage (mg)*
amobarbital	Amytal	Tablet: 30, 50, 100 mg	160–200
	Amytal Sodium	Capsule: 65, 200 mg	65–200
		Vial: 250, 500 mg	
aprobarbital	Atarate Alurate	Concentrate: 40 mg/5 ml (16-oz bottle)	5–20 ml
butabarbital†	Buticaps	Capsule: 15, 30 mg	50–100
	Butisol Sodium	Tablet: 15, 30, 50, 100 mg	50–100
		Concentrate: 30 mg/5 ml (16-oz bottle)	
pentobarbital	Nembutal	Capsule: 30, 50, 100 mg	100
		Concentrate: 20 mg/5 ml (16-oz bottle)	
		Parenteral: 50 mg/ml (2-ml ampule, 20- and 50-ml vials)	150–200
		Suppository: 30, 60, 120, 200 mg	120–200
phenobarbital	Generic	Capsule: 16, 65 mg (sustained release)	100–320
		Tablet: 8, 15, 16, 30, 32, 65, 100 mg	
		Concentrate: 16 mg/ml drops, 20 mg/5 ml	
		Parenteral: multiple strengths	100–320
secobarbital	Seconal	Capsule: 50, 100 mg	100
		Tablet: 100 mg	
		Parenteral: 50 mg/ml (20-ml vials, 1- and 2-ml syringes)	
secobarbital and amobarbital	Tuinal	Combinations of 25, 50, 100 mg each	50–200

Note. All of the above are believed to be available in generic form.
* Adult dosages. For child dosages, consult PDR or similar reference.
† Generic form available in tablets only.

at one or more key positions, resulting in differences in lipophilia and half-lives (see Figure 6-2).

The barbiturates have become less widely used because of their limited safety margin in overdosage, potential for dependence, and the degree of central nervous system depression they induce. These drugs are extremely potent hypnotics, particularly for patients who have not previously taken barbiturates. Indeed, some patients may demonstrate considerable somnolence 24 hours after ingestion. Moreover, these agents pose potential problems when mixed with alcohol or other central nervous system depressants and are contraindicated in patients with acute intermittent porphyria.

In depressed patients, the administration of barbiturates may result in a marked reduction of TCA plasma levels and diminutions of antidepressant effects because of their induction of liver microsomal enzymes and accelerated degradation of the tricyclic. Clinicians should keep this in mind when considering adjunctive usage of hypnotics in depressed patients. Indeed, we saw depressed patients chronically treated with barbiturates for sleep fail to respond to amitriptyline and other TCAs, but who did respond after discontinuing their barbiturates (see Chapter 9).

At present, the main remaining use in outpatient psychiatry for intermediate-acting sedative-hypnotic barbiturates, such as pentobarbital, is probably limited to the older patient who occasionally needs a hypnotic for insomnia and, because of prolonged past experience with barbiturates, finds a barbiturate sleeping pill preferable to any of the newer benzodiazepines. Such prescribing is of course a matter of giving in to a patient's experience and preference rather than a mandatory or necessary clinical maneuver. (For discussion of various uses of amobarbital—including for analytically oriented interviews—see Chapter 6.)

For patients who have become dependent on barbiturates, detoxification is necessary. Abrupt withdrawal should be avoided because it can result in seizures, delirium, and even death. When the daily dose of barbiturate is not known, physicians can give test doses of a barbiturate (watching for the emergence of nystagmus, slurred speech, ataxia, and sedation) to determine the currently needed dosage. This can then act as a barometer of the dose at which to begin a detoxification program (see Chapter 11).

SEDATIVE ANTIHISTAMINES

Hydroxyzine compounds are the only antihistamines with some documented efficacy in the treatment of anxiety disorders. They also enjoy indication for preoperative and postanesthesia sedation. These drugs are available in capsules or tablets ranging from 10 to 100 mg each. However, our clinical experience in psychiatric patients suggests that these drugs are neither much appreciated by patients nor particularly effective on the few occasions we have tried them. They are reasonably free of side effects, although hydroxyzine and the other antihistamines exert anticholinergic effects. When taken with other anticholinergic agents, hydroxyzine and related compounds can pose potential problems, particularly in high dosages. Their main value may be as a delaying action for patients who are inclined to abuse sedative-hypnotic or benzodiazepine drugs, since they do not produce either physical or psychic dependence.

Diphenhydramine (Benadryl) is another antihistamine that is sometimes used for its sedative or alleged hypnotic effects. It has not been well studied in either capacity but has some sedative properties and is occasionally judged by patients to be acceptable. Dosage for sleep is 50–100 mg. Diphenhydramine is now available over-the-counter in 25-mg forms. The drug is anticholinergic and can be used for acute dystonic reactions to antipsychotics (see Chapter 4). Promethazine (Phenergan) is a phenothiazine without antipsychotic properties that is marketed as an antihistamine with sedative properties. Again, it is occasionally found useful as a mild sedative at doses of 25–100 mg, but it is not a major psychiatric drug. Pyrilamine maleate, another antihistamine, is the ingredient that is used in most over-the-counter preparations (e.g., Compoz) that are used for either tranquilization or hypnosis.

Several TCAs exert marked antihistamine effects and are excellent hypnotics. Doxepin, amitriptyline, and trimipramine can be used in doses of 25–75 mg at bedtime. In an analysis of a major National Institute of Mental Health (NIMH) collaborative study, improved sleep in patients on a TCA was common but bore little relationship to overall clinical response, suggesting some tricyclics have hypnotic effects independent of their antidepressant activity.

"NONBARBITURATE" HYPNOTICS

In the late 1940s and the 1950s, several nonbarbiturate hypnotic drugs were developed in the hope that they would be safer and better than the barbiturates. Unfortunately, this hope was not realized. They proved, generally, to have as many limitations as the barbiturates. Only one of these currently available for use is generally viewed as safe and effective. This is chloral hydrate, which in doses between 500 and 1500 mg at bedtime is a somewhat effective and reasonably safe sleeping medication (Table 7-3 and Figure 7-2). Early prescription practices of 500 mg at sleep often proved inadequate to produce sedation, and most prescribers have come to favor 1,000 mg, particularly in younger adult patients. The drug is often used in double-blind trials of other psychiatric medications as an adjunct medication because of its presumed safety and "cleanliness." It is hard to tell whether this reputation is fully deserved, particularly since chloral hydrate itself was once widely abused in England in the early 1900s.

Another hypnotic, paraldehyde, is a colorless liquid with a very pungent odor and a burning, disagreeable taste. The

Table 7-3. Other nighttime hypnotic agents

Generic name	Brand name	Dosage forms	Dosage (mg)*
chloral hydrate†	Noctec	Capsule: 250, 500 mg Concentrate: 500 mg/ml (16-oz bottle)	500–1500
ethchlorvynol	Placidyl	Capsule: 100, 200, 500, 750 mg	500–750
ethinamate	Valmid	Capsule: 500 mg	500–1000
glutethimide	Doriden	Tablet: 250, 500 mg	250–500
methyprylon	Noludar	Tablet: 50, 200 mg	200–400
		Capsule: 300 mg	300

* Adult dosages. Patients may require slightly higher dosages of chloral hydrate or ethchlorvynol. For child dosages, consult PDR or similar reference.
† Available in generic form.

oral hypnotic dose is 5 or 10 ml. However, the medication has no advantages and may be quite toxic if the material is old and deteriorated. It is too irritating to be given parenterally, although intramuscular and rectal administration were once common. Paraldehyde's old place in the detoxification of chronic alcoholic patients is now supplanted by longer-acting and safer benzodiazepines.

Other "nonbarbiturate" hypnotics, including glutethimide, ethinamate, methyprylon, and ethchlorvynol, were developed because of the known dangers of addiction and lethality on suicidal ingestion of the barbiturates. Unfortunately, none of these drugs proved to be either safer or less capable of producing physical or psychic dependence than the drugs that they were supposed to replace. There are presently no logical reasons for using them in preference to the safer benzodiazepines.

METHAQUALONE

Methaqualone (Quaalude) still deserves some passing mention (Figure 7-2). This is the most recent of the nonbarbiturate

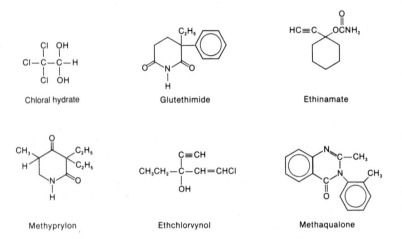

Figure 7-2. Chemical structures of nonbarbiturate hypnotics.

hypnotics marketed as a safe and effective replacement for the more dangerous older sleeping pills. It became widely abused in the illicit street market and achieved a good deal of publicity as the "love" drug in the 1960s. Methaqualone was alleged to have aphrodisiac properties, a proposition that has never been specifically tested in any scientific way. The drug, however, can cause paresthesias, which may somehow increase sexual feelings. It has acquired a remarkably tainted reputation and is now no longer available for prescription use. Whether the drug was really more likely to be abused or was more euphoriant than the barbiturates is quite unclear. The one available study relevant to the point suggested that it was really no different from pentobarbital in its subjective effects. In our local clinical experience in the past, we found occasional patients with severe insomnia who claimed methaqualone was far superior as a hypnotic—both in terms of speed of onset and lack of hangover—than other available hypnotics, even comparable barbiturates. In any event, methaqualone, for good or for bad, is no longer available.

L-TRYPTOPHAN

A hypnotic drug that seems to be free from dependence or abuse liability is the amino acid L-tryptophan. It has not been formally approved for medical use as a hypnotic drug in the United States but is available in both drug stores and health food stores as a dietary supplement either in the pure form or combined with other nutriments. There is reasonable evidence that, at doses of 1–6 g at bedtime, L-tryptophan has some efficacy as a sleeping pill in some patients with insomnia. It is neither as powerful as the major hypnotics nor, presumably, as dangerous. It is, however, a rather expensive way to get a night's sleep, since the drug costs almost $1 per g under most circumstances.

Starting dose should be 1–2 g at bedtime with an increase to 3–4 g after two to three nights. The amount of available L-tryptophan in milk—particularly when warmed—rivals a 2-g dose, and some clinicians have advocated this time-honored approach for insomnia. Some workers have further noted that carbohydrates facilitate the absorption of L-tryptophan, suggesting that milk and cookies may be better than milk alone. We know of no double-blind studies of this, however.

The ill-considered use of L-tryptophan for patients with insomnia or who are being treated with fluoxetine or MAOIs should be avoided. The serotonin syndrome manifested by myoclonic jerks, hyperpyrexia, confusion, and coma can be precipitated if doses of 1–4 g are given initially to patients on fluoxetine or MAOIs. The manufacturer of fluoxetine notes that the addition of L-tryptophan to the regimen of patients already being treated with fluoxetine is contraindicated. It is unclear whether beginning with 500 mg of L-tryptophan at bedtime and titrating upward is clinically useful or safe in patients on MAOIs. We have tried L-tryptophan in MAOI-related insomnia in doses of 1–2 g at bedtime with little success.

In 1989, a small series of seriously ill patients with fever, myalgia, and massive eosinophilia were identified. All had exposure to L-tryptophan, and most had persistent illness requiring steroids for relief. On this basis, the FDA withdrew all L-tryptophan from the market. It is currently only available as an investigational new drug or by order from Canadian pharmacies. If the presumed toxic ingredient is identified, the substance may again become available. The risk of the serious disease is unknown, but L-tryptophan was used for years without massive eosinophilia being seen.

Bibliography

Dement W, Seidel W, Carskadon M, et al: Changes in daytime sleepiness/alertness with nighttime benzodiazepines, in Pharmacology of Benzodiazepines. Edited by Usdin E, Skolnick P, Tallman JF, et al. New York, Macmillan, 1982, pp 219–228

Falco M: Methaqualone misuse: foreign experience and US drug control policy. Int J Addict 11:597–610, 1976

Gillin JC, Reynolds CF, Shipley JE: Sleep studies in selected adult neuropsychiatric disorders, in Psychiatry Update: American Psychiatric Association Annual Review, Vol 4. Edited by Hales RE, Frances AJ. Washington, DC, American Psychiatric Press, 1985, pp 352–360

Greenblatt DJ, Shader RI, Abernethy DR: Current status of benzodiazepines [first of two parts]. N Engl J Med 309:354–359, 1983

Greenblatt DJ, Shader RI, Abernethy DR: Current status of benzodiazepines [second of two parts]. N Engl J Med 309:410–415, 1983

Hertzman PA, Blevins WL, Mayer J, et al: Association of the eosinophilia-myalgia syndrome with the ingestion of tryptophan. N Engl J Med 322:869–873, 1990

Kales A: Benzodiazepines in the treatment of insomnia, in Pharmacology of Benzodiazepines. Edited by Usdin E, Skolnick P, Tallman JF, et al. New York, Macmillan, 1982, pp 199–217

Kales A: Quazepam: hypnotic efficacy and side effects. Pharmacotherapy 10:1–12, 1990

Katz MM, Koslow SH, Maas JW, et al: The timing, specificity and clinical prediction of tricyclic drug effects in depression. Psychol Med 17:297–309, 1987

Roffwarg H, Erman M: Evaluation and diagnosis of the sleep disorders: implications for psychiatry and other clinical specialties, in Psychiatry Update: American Psychiatric Association Annual Review, Vol 4. Edited by Hales RE, Frances AJ. Washington, DC, American Psychiatric Press, 1985, pp 294–328

Seidel WF, Roth T, Roehrs T, et al: Treatment of a 12 hour shift of sleep schedule with benzodiazepines. Science 224:1262–1264, 1985

Stimulants

The main available stimulant drugs with some evidence for utility in psychiatric conditions are *d*-amphetamine, methylphenidate, and magnesium pemoline, although a number of other amphetamine-like substances are marketed for use in weight reduction (Table 8-1). In addition, one interesting anorexiant, fenfluramine, is not a stimulant and probably does not deserve to be classified as an amphetamine but may have some minor uses in psychiatric conditions (e.g., infantile autism). Because of its effects on serotonergic function, one form of fenfluramine has been used as a challenge test in psychiatric research. The use of stimulants in psychiatric practice was reviewed extensively elsewhere (Chiarello and Cole 1987; Satel and Nelson 1989).

Amphetamine, originally available as a racemic amphetamine preparation, was in fact the first nonbarbiturate drug to be clinically effective in modern psychopharmacology. It was developed in the late 1930s and studied in children with severe behavior disorders, a condition originally called hyperactivity or minimal brain dysfunction, and more recently

Table 8-1. Stimulants

Generic name	Brand name	Preparations
d-amphetamine*	Dexedrine	Tablet: 5, 10 mg
		Spansule: 5, 10, 15 mg
		Elixir: 5 mg/5 ml (16-oz bottle)
d-methamphetamine hydrochloride	Desoxyn	Tablet: 5 mg
		Slow-release tablet: 5, 10, 15 mg
methylphenidate*	Ritalin	Tablet: 5, 10, 20 mg
		Slow-release tablet: 20 mg
magnesium pemoline	Cylert	Tablet: 18.75, 37.5, 75 mg
		Chewable tablet: 37.5 mg

*Available in generic form.

and more accurately classified in DSM-III-R as attention-deficit hyperactivity disorder (ADHD). In this condition, all three drugs—d-amphetamine, methylphenidate, and magnesium pemoline—are clearly more effective than placebo. The dose for d-amphetamine is 5–40 mg a day, for methylphenidate 10–80 mg a day, and for magnesium pemoline 18.75–150 mg per day.

These three drugs probably act by releasing dopamine into the synapse and may or may not also have direct agonist activity. They also have noradrenergic actions. In laboratory animals they increase motor activity and at very high doses produce repetitive "compulsive" behavior, including sniffing, staring, and paw-chewing. All three drugs tend to increase pulse rate and to a lesser extent blood pressure in high doses, and they tend to decrease appetite and to interfere with sleep. d-Amphetamine and methylphenidate, but not magnesium pemoline, are self-administered intravenously by laboratory animals and are well known to have abuse liability in humans. The major abuse of stimulants has been in the form of methamphetamine, which was used intravenously in very high doses during the flower-child period of the 1960s, resulting in heavily dependent individuals known as "speed freaks." Such individuals usually took the medication in relatively large doses in runs of a few days and then crashed for a day or two before starting again. Patterns of oral abuse were less intense and dramatic.

There has been a recent reemergence of methamphetamine abuse. The original formulation was the hydrochloride and was known as "speed." Crystalline methamphetamine base, known as "ice," is widely abused in Hawaii. It is chiefly smoked but is also used intravenously, the preferred route during the 1960s. When smoked, it appears to give a "rush" similar to cocaine but with a longer duration of the euphoric state. This fits with the known relative pharmacokinetics: methamphetamine should be metabolized more slowly than cocaine. In monkeys, cocaine is more "abusable" intravenously; they will work harder and longer to get cocaine and will continue self-administration for days without stopping, until death occurs. In contrast, amphetamines are less reinforcing. It is too early to tell whether smoked "ice" will be more or less of a problem than cocaine. Cho (1990) recently reviewed the pharmacology of "ice," but no studies and almost no other published reports on "ice" are available.

There is reasonable evidence that very high doses of *d*-amphetamine, generally over 80 mg a day and sometimes as high as 1,000–2,000 mg a day, can produce an acute psychosis that generally resembles paranoid schizophrenia but can occasionally present with delirium and other conventional signs of toxic drug psychosis. This condition is sometimes considered a model for schizophrenia or at least for acute paranoid psychosis. In addition, parenteral administration of methylphenidate has been used as a test to predict risk of psychotic relapse in schizophrenic patients.

Magnesium pemoline is a little different from the other two drugs, having a somewhat slower onset and offset of action, making it preferred in occasional patients who get symptom relief for 3 or 4 hours from a single dose of methylphenidate or *d*-amphetamine with an abrupt change in status as the drug wears off. In such patients, magnesium pemoline may be smoother and better tolerated. Child psychiatrists are concerned about hepatocellular damage due to magnesium pemoline and recommend a monthly check of liver function (see Chapter 12). We have not yet run into such a problem in adult patients. That magnesium pemoline prescriptions can be refilled and phoned in to pharmacies makes it the most flexible stimulant to use clinically.

d-Amphetamine and d-methamphetamine are both available in sustained-release forms. Some experienced clinicians believe that the methamphetamine sustained-release preparation (Desoxyn Gradumet tablets) delivers a more level and prolonged effect for 4–8 hours than the d-amphetamine spansules, which tend to produce an intense early effect that fades over the next several hours.

USES OF STIMULANTS

Attention-Deficit Hyperactivity Disorder

ADHD is the only condition other than narcolepsy and weight reduction for which stimulants are approved currently by the FDA. In children, the syndrome is manifested by very short attention span, overactivity, irritability, poor social relations, impulsivity, occasional angry or assaultive behavior, poor school performance, and apparent inability to benefit from instruction or limit setting. Some children with the syndrome have a parent with a history or current symptoms of a similar condition. Occasional children with the syndrome have clear evidence of central nervous system damage at birth or subsequently; the majority of such patients, however, do not have any clear evidence of "hard" neurological signs of clearly diagnosable brain injury or abnormality.

In children with ADHD, any of the three drugs are likely to be clinically better than placebo in about 70–80% of those treated; about 30% show a clear and highly impressive degree of clinical improvement, and another 40% show some modulation of behavior that may be of some clinical importance. Occasionally, children are made more active by these drugs. In the first weeks of treatment, children often look drawn and even somewhat depressed and rarely show any euphoriant effect from the medication. It is not clear that the drugs dramatically reduce activity level. They probably act by improving attention span and organizing behavior more effectively. Some degree of growth inhibition or weight loss has been reported in children, but these are generally not major problems. (See Chapter 12 for further discussion about use of stimulants in children.)

Wender et al. (1985) at the University of Utah, Huessey (1979) at the University of Vermont, and others have identified adults with symptoms resembling those seen in children with ADHD and have shown that such adults may respond to stimulant therapy. These drug responders are very likely to have been remembered as "hyperkinetic" children by their parents. Some individuals who have had clear clinical benefit from stimulants in childhood continue to require and to benefit from stimulant medication well into adult life. Many children with ADHD seem to grow out of the major manifestations of the illness at some time in adolescence, although they are often left with residual symptoms of impaired concentration or coping ability, which may or may not be benefited by further stimulant administration.

The interesting and clinically useful aspect of stimulant therapy in either children or adults with ADHD is that clinical effects are often clear and dramatic within a day or two of reaching the appropriate dosage. This stands in dramatic contrast to the more conventional antidepressants and antipsychotics, which often take days or even weeks to achieve a satisfactory clinical result.

In clinical practice, adults with personality disorder, short attention span, restlessness, hyperactivity, irritability, impulsivity, and related symptoms sometimes present with a history of illicit drug abuse. In such individuals, a trial of a stimulant raises an ethical problem: when it is clear that any stimulant will be abused, the drug cannot be used. Stimulants can be used in patients with a history of drug abuse under the following circumstances:

1. When the stimulant drug has clearly been used to improve functioning rather than to produce euphoria or to get "high"
2. When a good therapeutic alliance is available
3. When the medication can be closely monitored, perhaps in an inpatient setting
4. When other approaches have failed
5. When the patient's problems are seriously interfering with his or her life functioning

Some children and adults with ADHD respond to desipramine, and this can be used in patients who might abuse a stimulant. Bromocriptine is another drug that can be used in this situation.

Depression

In the early literature on the use of amphetamine in psychiatry, there were a number of case reports of individuals presenting with the full syndrome of endogenous depression who responded dramatically to racemic amphetamine. There have been a few double-blind trials completed at one time or another over the past 30 years that show some evidence of clinical efficacy of stimulants in depressed outpatients. Not all studies are positive; some are only weakly positive and some are clearly negative.

Given the bad repute into which stimulants have fallen, it is probably not reasonable to conduct further trials of stimulants in fresh non-treatment-resistant depressed patients. However, in patients with chronic treatment-resistant depression that has failed to respond to a range of standard antidepressants, stimulants will occasionally provide excellent symptomatic relief and will enable the patient to function adequately for prolonged periods without side effects and without any indication that the drug is being abused or misused. Some of these patients have clear endogenous symptoms, others appear to have atypical depressions of one sort or another, and still others have major symptoms of fatigue or neurasthenia. It is not possible to tell in advance which depressed patients will benefit. Rickels et al. (1970) suggested some time ago that relatively heavy intake of coffee (four cups a day or more) was a predictor of good clinical response, at least to magnesium pemoline. In contrast, patients who are intolerant of caffeine often cannot tolerate stimulants. However, experience at McLean Hospital suggests that some depressed patients with excellent response to stimulants dislike or avoid caffeine-containing beverages.

Stimulants also have a place in the crisis management of individuals whose functioning is impaired by depression and whose life situation will deteriorate rapidly if they are not able to resume functioning within a few days. In such situations a trial of methylphenidate, *d*-amphetamine, or magnesium pemoline is worth initiating to attempt to get a patient through a crisis period where failure to function might result in getting fired from a job or flunking out of college.

In such situations the clinician may well begin with magnesium pemoline because it is the least abusable of the stimulants and also because it can be prescribed by telephone and prescriptions can be refilled, options not available with *d*-amphetamine or methylphenidate, which are Class II drugs. A good initial dose of magnesium pemoline is 37.5 mg to be given in the morning with a repeat dose in the early afternoon if the initial dose is helpful. If the dose is overstimulating, half a tablet (18.75 mg) can be tried instead. If the dose has no appreciable effect, it can be doubled or even tripled in the morning and again later in the day as needed, up to 75 mg twice a day. Usually within a few days it is clear whether the patient has had a distinct improvement in mental status and functioning. Patients should be advised that if the drug is unpleasantly stimulating or produces any undesirable side effects, they should stop taking it at once and contact their physician. If magnesium pemoline is ineffective or if the patient finds it either sedative or oddly dysphoric, then methylphenidate or d-amphetamine may work instead. With these drugs, doses up to 20 or 30 mg of d-amphetamine a day or twice that amount of methylphenidate can be tried.

Some patients will show an initial excellent response to a stimulant medication and then develop rapid tolerance and lose all effect, whereas others will go on and continue to benefit from the same low dose of the stimulant for months or even years. Other patients feel anxious, agitated, and unpleasantly "wired" on some or all stimulants. If the drug is to be stopped, it can be either tapered or stopped abruptly. Some rebound depression may occur (see Chapter 11). Patients with a history of pronounced mood disturbances may require hospitalization.

d-Amphetamine is available in 5-, 10-, and 15-mg spansule (slow-release) formulations. Methamphetamine (Desoxyn Gradumet tablets) is available in 5-, 10-, and 15-mg slow-release tablets. Some patients prefer taking ordinary tablets of d-amphetamine or methylphenidate and may take the whole day's dose at once on arising, even if 30 or 40 mg a day is being given. Such patients feel no rush or high but are relieved of depression for at least 24 hours. Others take single fast-release tablets several times a day, taking another as the effect of the first dose wears off. Some dislike this on-off effect and prefer sustained-release preparations.

Phenylpropanolamine is marketed as an over-the-counter antiobesity pill in 37.5-mg and 75-mg dosage strengths, usually in a sustained-release preparation. We have seen occasional patients with either depression or ADHD who have found phenylpropanolamine helpful in the way a standard stimulant sometimes is. However, most patients and most recreational drug users find the subjective effects of phenylpropanolamine mildly unpleasant. When phenyl-propanolamine was abused in "triple threat" illicit pills containing ephedrine and caffeine as well, it is likely that the ephedrine or the combination accounted for the pills' amphetamine-like properties. Phenylpropanolamine alone may reduce appetite and increase pulse and blood pressure a little but is not a useful stimulant. It should be noted that the drug marketed in Europe as phenylpropanolamine is, in fact, a different stereoisomer and does have amphetamine-like stimulant effects.

Acquired immunodeficiency syndrome (AIDS). Patients with AIDS often have a mixture of depression, fatigue, and difficulty initiating activities, perhaps a form of akinesia. Such patients may have central nervous system complications of AIDS including shrinking of the basal ganglia. Standard tricyclic antidepressants tend to be poorly tolerated and may cause increased memory problems or delirium. Methylphenidate appears to be widely used in such patients with excellent results, though little has been written about this use. Patients can be started on low doses (e.g., 5 mg bid) titrated to the relief of symptoms in the absence of side effects. The dose may need to be increased gradually as the disease progresses. Local experts in Boston give us the impression that methylphenidate in AIDS-related depression, inertia, and confusion resembles L-dopa in parkinsonism, a replacement therapy needed because of changes in the brain. This idea is, of course, pure speculation. Other stimulants have not, to our knowledge, been tried in AIDS patients, but there is no obvious reason why *d*-amphetamine, *d*-methamphetamine, or pemoline should not be tried. Some children with ADHD do better on one than another, and stimulant-responsive depressed patients often have clearly better responses to one of these drugs than to the others for no known reason.

Other medical conditions.   A growing series of case reports document the usefulness of stimulants in patients on the medical wards of general hospitals. These patients have various combinations of debilitating depression and fatigue, which make them unable to cooperate in necessary treatments, and they lose weight rapidly. In this situation, standard antidepressants simply do not have a fast-enough onset of action. Stimulants do, probably about 50% of the time. They are therefore used more commonly and are helpful and appear safe.

Drug combinations.   Methylphenidate and *d*-amphetamine both interact with imipramine in laboratory animals to potentiate response to electrical stimulation of pleasure centers. Part of this is pharmacokinetic in the sense that the stimulant and the tricyclic interfere with each other's metabolism causing higher blood levels of each. This property is sometimes used clinically when methylphenidate is prescribed early in tricyclic therapy to hasten response. If a patient improves on methylphenidate plus imipramine it is impossible to tell for sure whether the clinical response is due to 1) the methylphenidate alone, 2) a longer period on imipramine, 3) the elevation of imipramine blood level caused by methylphenidate, or 4) a true combined effect of the two drugs. Generally, we do not recommend this combination approach (see Chapter 9).

Intuitively, it should be considered clinically dangerous to combine a stimulant with a monoamine oxidase inhibitor (MAOI), since the addition of a stimulant *could* precipitate a hypertensive crisis. However, we know of a few patients who have, on their own responsibility, added magnesium pemoline, methylphenidate, *d*-amphetamine, or cocaine to reverse MAOI-induced sedation or lack of clinical response, with alleged good subjective effects and no apparent effect on blood pressure. Other such patients have been described in the literature. We have seen hypertensive crises when phenylpropanolamine was added to an MAOI, but so far we have not encountered any with stimulant-MAOI combinations. Stimulant-MAOI combinations are not recommended in general practice; however, the combination has been used cautiously to counteract MAOI-induced hypotension (see Chapter 3).

Psychosis

Although the older literature from the 1930s and 1940s on the use of racemic amphetamine, *d*-amphetamine, and methylphenidate in patients with what was then called chronic schizophrenia is mixed (some patients improved on stimulant given alone, some showed no change, and some worsened), more recent studies of single doses of intravenous methylphenidate show that it increases psychosis in acutely ill patients with manic or schizophrenic disorders but has only a mild stimulant effect when such patients are in remission. More recent studies by Angrist et al. (1980) and Lieberman et al. (1983) show that chronically ill schizophrenic outpatients who show increased psychosis after a single dose of a stimulant are much more likely to relapse into a psychotic exacerbation than are patients who show no worsening on stimulant administration.

Another drug, fenfluramine, chemically resembles amphetamine but pharmacologically has serotonergic rather than dopaminergic effects. It is available clinically for use in obesity and is generally sedative rather than stimulating. On the basis of local experience in a few patients, fenfluramine raises tricyclic blood levels substantially when given in 20–40 mg a day doses to patients who run very low tricyclic blood levels despite adequate oral doses (e.g., 300 mg of imipramine). We have tried adding fenfluramine to the drug regimen of psychiatric patients gaining excess weight on a variety of classes of drug in the hope that fenfluramine would promote weight reduction without aggravating psychosis or mania. (Fenfluramine was once studied in mania and had weak antimanic effects.) Unfortunately, fenfluramine has, so far, not fulfilled its theoretical promise as a "safe" anorexiant in psychiatric patients. It is safe but does not cause weight loss.

A series of articles have dealt with the use of fenfluramine in autism. The drug lowers blood serotonin levels, which are sometimes elevated in autism. So far the evidence suggests that some autistic patients function better on fenfluramine, those with higher IQs responding better. The original idea that patients with the higher blood serotonin levels respond best appears to be incorrect, but there is some relation between the observed decrease in blood serotonin and response. There is a suggestion, however, that long-term fenfluramine exposure may cause neurotoxicity in laboratory animals. This area was reviewed by Biederman (1985).

Use Versus Abuse

We occasionally have seen patients who have, in the past, taken prescribed stimulants for years with claimed excellent relief of depression, fatigue, or disorganized behavior and have been taken off the drug by a physician concerned about "drug abuse." Such patients often have then failed to respond to a variety of more conventional tricyclic antidepressants and have been dysphoric and unable to function adequately for years. When the stimulant is represcribed, these patients often do quite well again for prolonged periods. It may be very hard to tell whether such individuals (who rarely have histories suggestive of ADHD) really have a uniquely stimulant-responsive disorder or whether they somehow have become "dependent" on stimulants. Either way, if they cope well and feel well only on stimulants, take low to moderate dosages as prescribed, and do not develop tolerance, the stimulant should be continued. If the physician feels uncomfortable about prescribing stimulants in such patients, consultation with a clinical psychopharmacologist may provide helpful clinical and ethical support.

More difficult permutations of the problem exist, of course. What about a patient who recalls *d*-amphetamine as making him feel "better" but not better enough to actually complete graduate courses or even to motivate him to pay the bill of the psychiatrist who was prescribing the pills? What about a patient who has failed on a host of antidepressants but refuses to try an MAOI because of the restricted diet and risks? Should she be forced to fail on an MAOI before a stimulant is tried or retried? What about a marginally employed, vague, mildly paranoid young man with severe ear pain of an undiagnosable nature who buys illicit stimulants to relieve the pain? The stimulants do not help him function, they do not make him more paranoid—they only make him feel better. What about the chronically very depressed woman who only feels better on 200 mg of methylphenidate a day?

We feel more comfortable prescribing stimulants when they either obviously improve functioning or when they at least relieve incapacitating distress. We would not force a patient to try an MAOI if he or she has already improved on a stimulant in the past, but these are personal judgments.

In summary, we suspect that the useful, rapidly acting stimulant drugs are underutilized in American psychiatry—they do not always work or even help, but when they do they can be very effective. It is too early to tell whether bupropion, which resembles the stimulants in some respects (see Chapter 3), will provide a safer, less abusable drug that will help those psychiatric patients who now only respond to standard stimulants.

Bibliography

Angrist B, Rotrosen J, Gershon S: Responses to apomorphine, amphetamine, and neuroleptics in schizophrenic subjects. Psychopharmacology 67:31–38, 1980

Angrist B, Peselow E, Rubinstein M, et al: Amphetamine response and relapse risk after depot neuroleptic discontinuation. Psychopharmacology 85:277–283, 1985

August GJ, Naftali R, Papanicolaou AC, et al: Fenfluramine treatment in infantile autism: neurochemical electrophysiological and behavioral effects. J Nerv Ment Dis 172:604–612, 1984

Biederman G: Fenfluramine (Pondimin) in autism. Biological Therapies in Psychiatry 8:25–28, 1985

Chiarello RJ, Cole JO: The use of psychostimulants in general psychiatry: a reconsideration. Arch Gen Psychiatry 44:286–295, 1987

Cho AK: Ice: a new dosage form of an old drug. Science 249:631–634, 1990

Cole JO (ed): The amphetamines in psychiatry. Seminars in Psychiatry 1:128–137, 1969

Cole JO: Drug therapy of adult minimal brain dysfunction, in Psychopharmacology Update. Edited by Cole JO. Lexington, MA, Collamore Press, 1981, pp 69–80

Davidoff E, Reifenstein E: Treatment of schizophrenia with sympathomimetic drugs: benzedrine sulfate. Psychiatr Q 13:127–144, 1939

Elizur A, Wintner I, Davidson S: The clinical and psychological effects of pemoline in depressed patients—a controlled study. International Pharmacopsychiatry 14:127–134, 1979

Ellinwood EH: Amphetamine psychosis: individuals, settings, and sequences, in Current Concepts on Amphetamine Abuse (DHEW Publ No HSM-729085). Edited by Ellinwood EH, Cohen S. Washington, DC, U.S. Government Printing Office, pp 143–158

Feighner JP, Herbstein J, Damlouji N: Combined MAOI, TCA, and direct stimulant therapy of treatment-resistant depression. J Clin Psychiatry 46:206–209, 1985

Fernandez F, Levy JK, Galizzi H: Response of HIV-related depression to psychostimulants: case reports. Hosp Community Psychiatry 39:628–631, 1988

Huessey H: Clinical explorations in adult MBD, in Psychiatric Aspects of Minimal Brain Dysfunction in Adults. Edited by Bellak L. New York, Grune & Stratton, 1979

Jackson JG: Hazards of smokable methamphetamine. N Engl J Med 321:907, 1989

Kaufmann M, Murray G, Cassem N: Use of psychostimulants in medically ill depressed patients. Psychosomatics 23:817–819, 1982

Klein R, Mannuzza S: Hyperactive boys almost grown up, III: methylphenidate effects on ultimate height. Arch Gen Psychiatry 45:1131–1134, 1988

Lieberman J, Kane J, Gadaletta D, et al: The use of methylphenidate challenge test as a predictor of relapse in schizophrenia. Paper presented at the American Psychiatric Association meeting, New York, May 5, 1983

Myerson A: The effect of benzedrine sulfate on mood and fatigue in normal and neurotic persons. AMA Archives of Neurology and Psychiatry 36:816–822, 1936

Rickels K, Gordon P, Gansman D, et al: Pemoline and methylphenidate in mildly depressed outpatients. Clin Pharmacol Ther 11:698–710, 1970

Ritvo ER, Freeman BJ, Yuwiler A: Study of fenfluramine in outpatients with the syndrome of autism. J Pediatr 105:823–828, 1984

Satel S, Nelson JC: Stimulants in the treatment of depression: a critical overview. J Clin Psychiatry 50:241–249, 1989

Wender PH, Reimherr FW, Wood D, et al: A controlled study of methylphenidate in the treatment of attention deficit disorder, residual type in adults. Am J Psychiatry 142:547–552, 1985

Wood DR, Reinherr FW, Wender PH, et al: Diagnosis and treatment of minimal brain dysfunction in adults: a preliminary report. Arch Gen Psychiatry 33:1453–1460, 1976

Combination and Adjunctive Treatments

9

It is the general hope of all clinicians that patients will respond to a single psychotherapeutic agent. However, this may be the exception rather than the rule. Although there has been much warranted consternation regarding polypharmacy (patients receiving too many different types of medications), some patients do require simultaneous treatment with different classes of drugs. Until more is learned about the biochemistry of various disorders and the range of pharmacologic effects of available and future medications, clinicians will constantly be faced with using more than one agent to effect a positive response in individual patients. Obviously, the number of potential combinations is vast and beyond the scope of this chapter. We recommend that clinicians become familiar with a number of commonly used combination drugs or combination regimens that have been reported in recent years to be particularly effective in specific clinical situations. In addition, clinicians should become familiar with combinations that can pose potential difficulties because of drug-drug interactions or additive side effects.

(The use of antiparkinsonians and benzodiazepines in combination with neuroleptics is discussed in detail in Chapter 4; other possible combinations are discussed throughout the text.)

AMITRIPTYLINE-PERPHENAZINE

Amitriptyline, a tricyclic antidepressant (TCA), is marketed in combination with a phenothiazine antipsychotic, perphenazine. This combination appears under two trade names: Triavil and Etrafon (Table 9-1). Various combinations of strengths are available, and these are coded according to the dose of each drug contained in the capsule; the dosage of perphenazine is given first. For example, a capsule of Triavil or Etrafon 2-25 contains 2 mg of perphenazine and 25 mg of amitriptyline (Table 9-1). This neuroleptic-tricyclic combination is widely used in the United States and is generally prescribed by primary-care practitioners. However, experienced psychopharmacologists advocate prescribing each drug individually to allow for optimum flexibility in dosing.

The indications for this combination are anxiety and agitation associated with depression in both neurotic and psychotic patients, including those with schizophrenia and physical disease. Theoretically and practically, these agents might best be used to treat patients with psychotic depression, an illness that often responds more favorably to this combination or electroconvulsive therapy than to tricyclics alone. This preferential response suggests a possible involvement of dopaminergic systems in delusional depression.

One major issue that has arisen is whether the combination's preferential benefit in delusional depression is due to its combined pharmacologic effects rather than to the higher blood levels of amitriptyline produced by simultaneous administration of a phenothiazine and vice versa; each drug elevates the blood level of the other. (See the section "Tricyclic Blood Levels" in Chapter 3.) Data from double-blind studies

Table 9-1. Combination antidepressants

Generic name	Brand name	Dosage forms*	Dosage schedule (mg)†
chlordiazepoxide + amitriptyline	Limbitrol	Tablet: 5–12.5, 10–25 mg	To start: 3–4/day of 10–25 mg tabs then 2–6/day as needed
perphenazine + amitriptyline	Etrafon	Tablet: 2–10, 2–25, 4–10, 4–25 mg	To start: 1 2–25 or 4–25 tid or qid up to 8/day of any strength
	Triavil	Tablet: 2–10, 2–25, 4–10, 4–25, 4–50 mg	To start: 1 2–25 or 4–25 tid or qid or 1 4–50 with increases to a maximum of 4 4–50/day or 8/day of other strengths

*Dosage forms list amount (in milligrams) of first and second ingredients, respectively.
†Adult dosages. Some patients may require lower dosages.

by Spiker et al. (1985) comparing perphenazine, amitriptyline, and the combination in delusional depression suggest that the additive pharmacologic properties of the combination are of paramount importance rather than enhanced tricyclic or neuroleptic blood levels. However, the relatively higher TCA plasma levels attained with such combination drugs could help explain the results of early studies that showed reasonable antidepressant efficacy in nondelusional depressed patients using combinations that contained relatively low doses of the tricyclic. Conceivably, in those early studies, patients responded because they were attaining relatively higher TCA plasma levels than they would if prescribed a TCA alone.

Amitriptyline-perphenazine will produce greater anticholinergic effects than amitriptyline alone because of increased plasma levels as well as additive anticholinergic effects.

Fortunately, perphenazine produces relatively limited anticholinergic side reactions, making this less of an issue than for other potential combinations of phenothiazines and amitriptyline. For example, of the neuroleptics, thioridazine produces the most pronounced anticholinergic side effects and when added to amitriptyline—the most potent anticholinergic of the tricyclics—can result in marked anticholinergic reactions. This combination should obviously be used with caution.

The manufacturer's recommended starting dose of Triavil is one 2-25 or 4-25 tablet three times per day or two 4-50 tablets per day. The maintenance dose is two to four tablets per day. For elderly and adolescent patients, the recommended starting dose is one 4-10 Triavil tablet three times per day. We recommend that clinicians opt for prescribing the components of amitriptyline-perphenazine compounds individually to allow for increased flexibility. This is particularly important so as to avoid extended exposure to phenothiazine. Long-term use of phenothiazines can result in tardive dyskinesia, which has been reported as possibly being more common in patients with major affective disorders than in those with schizophrenia (see Chapter 4).

CHLORDIAZEPOXIDE-AMITRIPTYLINE

The combination of amitriptyline and chlordiazepoxide was introduced in the United States in 1980 and marketed under the brand name of Limbitrol (Table 9-1). It carries an FDA-approved indication for the treatment of patients with mixed anxiety and depression. The numerical designation parallels that of Triavil. Limbitrol 10-25 contains 10 mg of chlordiazepoxide and 25 mg of amitriptyline. It is also available in a 5-12.5 form (Table 9-1). The recommended starting dose in adults is three to four tablets per day of the 10-25 strength with a recommended maximum daily dose of six tablets per day. In elderly patients, the recommended starting dose is one 5-12.5 tablet three or four times a day.

Although data from previous studies indicate that chlordiazepoxide alone is not an effective antidepressant, the combination has been shown to decrease anxiety, to aid sleep early in treatment (within the first 2 weeks), and to be associated with better patient compliance. However, published studies do not indicate that continued additional benefit can be obtained after the initial 4–6 weeks. Wherever possible, clinicians who have used the combination for this initial period should consider switching to prescribing these agents individually and eventually tapering the benzodiazepine.

There are considerable differences between combinations of amitriptyline with perphenazine and those with chlordiazepoxide. Enhanced efficacy of the chlordiazepoxide-amitriptyline combination early in treatment is not due to any increase in TCA plasma levels, since benzodiazepines, unlike antipsychotics, do not usually slow microsomal enzymatic activity in the liver. (However, since chlordiazepoxide does not increase TCA plasma levels, six 10-25 tablets per day may produce an inadequate TCA blood level for many seriously depressed patients.) The benzodiazepines are not anticholinergic and do not pose a problem in this regard. They can, however, add to the sedation produced by amitriptyline alone. In our experience, it is rarely necessary to add a benzodiazepine to amitriptyline early in treatment.

OTHER ANTIDEPRESSANT-BENZODIAZEPINE COMBINATIONS

Three recent studies indicate that specific benzodiazepines may interact with some antidepressants to produce higher plasma levels of either drug. Lemberger et al. (1988) recently reported that fluoxetine may increase plasma levels of diazepam. In another report (The Upjohn Company 1990), 80 normal male volunteers received one of four drug regimens per day for 4 days: 4 mg of alprazolam, 60 mg of fluoxetine combined with 4 mg of alprazolam, 60 mg of fluoxetine, or placebo. The combination of fluoxetine and alprazolam produced approximately a 30% increase in plasma alprazolam levels compared with alprazolam alone. Psychomotor decrements over alprazolam alone were noted with the combination but were not thought to warrant adjustment in dosage of either drug. Fluoxetine and norfluoxetine blood levels were not increased with the combination. Although it is difficult to extrapolate from this study to clinical use, it does suggest more careful monitoring should be instituted when fluoxetine is combined with a benzodiazepine.

In another study (The Upjohn Company 1986), patients with major depression who had been maintained on imipramine were started on alprazolam, which was increased to 4 mg over 10 days, maintained for 7 days, and then tapered over 15 days. Imipramine and desipramine levels increased approximately 30% during alprazolam dosing. Generally, patients improved with the combination without an increase in side effects. No placebo control was used. Again, it is difficult to determine the clinical significance of these observations; however, they suggest that earlier reports that some benzodiazepines do not increase plasma levels of TCAs cannot be generalized. Rather, clinicians should keep this in mind when prescribing the combination and be aware of possible benefits and side effects.

L-TRIIODOTHYRONINE-TCA COMBINATIONS

A number of years ago a debate emerged in the literature as to whether thyroid preparations (e.g., L-triiodothyronine [T_3]) when prescribed with a TCA hastened the speed of onset of the antidepressant effect: Early studies in women suggested it did, although later studies in men, which also employed higher dosages of tricyclics, failed to substantiate the early finding. Then, a fallow period followed for this combination until 1982, when Goodwin et al. reported that the addition of 25–50 μg/day of T_3 (Cytomel) brought out within 7 days a clinical response in patients who had previously not responded to a seemingly adequate TCA trial. A number of subsequent clinical reports have confirmed this observation, although some clinicians have reported responses requiring 7–10 days of combined therapy. We believe it is reasonable to add 25 μg/day of T_3 for 7 days to a tricyclic before switching to another antidepressant. This can be further increased to 37.5 μg or 50 μg for an additional week if only a limited change is seen at day 7. Generally, patients experience few additional side effects, although we have occasionally seen patients complain of headaches or of feeling warm. If a patient responds positively, we recommend continuing the T_3 for an additional 60 days and then tapering by 12.5 μg every 3 days. Some patients will demonstrate a resumption of symptoms and will require reinstitution of the T_3. One of our patients required resumption of dose and maintenance for more than 1 year before finally able to be tapered off T_3. Thyroid function tests while the patient was on T_3 were essentially normal. After tapering, T_3 uptake, thyroid-stimulating hormone (TSH), and levothyroxine (T_4) were all lower than normal, but normalized within 2–3 weeks. This patient demonstrated none of the stigmata of decreased thyroid status immediately after discontinuation.

Overall, it is our impression that Cytomel (T_3) is most useful in patients with pronounced psychomotor retardation. We have on occasion found that it can also bring out a response in patients who have relapsed while on a tricyclic to which they had previously responded.

The mechanism of action of T_3 potentiation of tricyclics is undetermined. Generally, theories have revolved around its facilitating receptor adaptation. However, Targum et al. (1983) reported that T_3 responders had demonstrated relatively enhanced thyroid-stimulating hormone responses to thyrotropin-releasing hormone infusions, suggesting that a subtle form of thyroid dysfunction might play a role in these patients.

Clinicians frequently ask whether Synthroid (T_4) is as effective as T_3 in augmenting response to TCAs. T_4 is metabolized to T_3 in humans. A recent double-blind study comparing 2-week treatments of T_4 and T_3 indicated that T_3 is significantly more effective. However, since T_4 has a much longer half-life, patients may not have achieved steady state on T_4, leaving conclusions open to question (Joffe and Singer 1987).

LITHIUM-TCA COMBINATIONS

Lithium has been well studied in its own right as an antidepressant. Overall, the drug is effective in some 50% of patients, with suggestions that it is best used in males with bipolar depression (see Chapters 3 and 5). de Montigny et al. (1981, 1983) reported that the addition of lithium carbonate to a tricyclic trial resulted in clinical improvement within 7–14 days in patients who had failed to respond to a TCA alone. These observations have been confirmed in two double-blind studies. Response is often at low dosages (600–1,200 mg/day) and at low serum levels (<0.8 meq/L). The mechanism of action has been hypothesized as a potentiation of serotonergic activity—either via increased biosynthesis or receptor adaptation. Our experience with the combination has been generally favorable, and we have been particularly impressed with results obtained in depressed patients with pronounced obsessionality and agitation. Price et al. (1983) reported that lithium carbonate also elicited a response in patients with delusional depression who had not responded to amitriptyline-perphenazine alone.

Lithium may also augment responses to other antidepressants. For example, bipolar depressed patients with hypersomnia and hyperphagia (previously termed "atypical") may respond dramatically to the combination of lithium with the monoamine oxidase inhibitor (MAOI) tranylcypromine. In addition, lithium has been combined successfully with fluoxetine (Pope et al. 1988).

In a New Haven follow-up study, unipolar depressed patients treated with desipramine plus lithium remained euthymic in the community when off medication for much longer periods than did patients who improved on desipramine plus placebo (Nierenberg et al. 1990). For further discussion of maintenance treatment, see Chapter 5.

Overall, we would not expect more than 50% of TCA nonresponders to respond to the addition of either T_3 (Cytomel) or lithium carbonate. The clinician should strongly consider either one of these strategies before switching to other antidepressants. If lithium carbonate is to be added, it should be initiated at 300 mg twice a day for 2 days and increased to 900 mg/day for 3–4 days with a further increase to 1,200 mg/day for a total 10- to 14-day trial.

METHYLPHENIDATE-TCA COMBINATIONS

In the early 1970s, Wharton and colleagues reported that the addition of methylphenidate increased plasma levels of tricyclics by inhibiting microsomal degradation of the TCA in the liver (similar to that observed with antipsychotic agents). This approach offers a possible way of increasing TCA plasma levels without increasing the dose of the TCA. In addition to this effect, methylphenidate is a stimulant and may be useful in treating the anergia and psychomotor retardation of endogenous depression. However, as described in the previous chapter, we do not recommend adding methylphenidate for increasing plasma levels, because clinicians can attain higher TCA plasma levels by increasing TCA dosages themselves. Rather, clinicians might want to use methylphenidate for its energizing properties but should keep in mind it may increase TCA plasma levels and side effects.

BETHANECHOL-TCA COMBINATIONS

The anticholinergic effects of the TCAs can be severe (see Chapter 3). Peripherally these include dry mouth, heartburn secondary to esophageal reflux, constipation, urinary hesitance or inability to void, and blurred vision. Central nervous system effects include problems with memory, speech blockage, confusion, and visual hallucinosis.

Peripheral anticholinergic effects may be ameliorated via the introduction of bethanechol (Urecholine)—a cholinergic agonist—in doses ranging between 50 and 200 mg/day. It is usually given as 25 mg tid or qid, increasing the dose to 50 mg tid or qid if neither improvement nor cholinergic side effects (e.g., abdominal cramps) occur; side effects are uncommon. Originally reported in an open study by Everett in 1976, its use, to our knowledge, has not been assessed under double-blind conditions. Our experience has been that bethanechol is more helpful for urinary hesitance than for constipation and blurred vision but that overall it is of limited efficacy. The acute use of bethanechol to aid patients who develop impotence on TCAs (25 mg taken an hour or so before attempting intercourse) has been advocated. Here, also, our limited experience has not been particularly favorable.

PHYSOSTIGMINE AS AN ANTICHOLINERGIC ANTIDOTE

When patients develop confusion on TCAs, antiparkinsonian agents, and antipsychotics, clinicians should consider anticholinergic delirium, a major problem when it occurs. This should be managed primarily with dose reduction or discontinuation. The parenteral administration of physostigmine—a cholinesterase inhibitor that crosses the blood-brain barrier—was at times used as a possible clinical test for anticholinergic delirium. The drug was administered in a single 0.5-cc (1.0 mg/cc) dose and could be repeated once after 20–

30 minutes if no effect was noted. Positive effects—clearing of confusion—often occurred rapidly, within 10–15 minutes.

Because physostigmine produced intense nausea and vomiting (either because of central or peripheral effects) and seizures, its use as a challenge test has waned greatly. At one time, some investigators advocated using physostigmine in combination with methscopolamine; however, this combination did not always block the emetic effects of the physostigmine, probably because they represent both central and peripheral effects.

MAOI-TCA COMBINATIONS

One of the most controversial combinations is MAOIs with TCAs. Although proscribed in *PDR*, the combination can be relatively safe and is occasionally effective in patients who have failed to respond to treatment with an MAOI or TCA alone. As indicated in Chapter 3, MAOIs when prescribed with sympathomimetic agents can result in acute hypertensive crises. Since TCAs exert an effect on sympathetic systems, prudence is warranted. Early fears of the combination came largely from a number of deaths that resulted from overdosages of the combination. However, overdosages of either TCAs or MAOIs alone can be lethal.

In contrast to these reports, some clinicians have argued that the combination can be of unique benefit. However, double-blind studies comparing a TCA, an MAOI, and their combination in non-treatment-resistant depressed patients have failed to show that the combination is of added benefit. However, the combination also does not appear to be more dangerous. Indeed, recent studies in humans and in animals suggest that some tricyclics may protect against hypertensive crises, although they may not afford protection against hyperpyrexic reactions.

The lack of superior efficacy for the MAOI-TCA combination could reflect the limited dosages of both drugs used—

e.g., 45 mg of phenelzine and 150 mg of amitriptyline. Some investigators have reported to us that combining higher dosages of both is effective, and we have noted positive results in some patients. However, generally speaking, a number of important caveats should be noted: 1) It appears safest to start the two drugs together. Adding the TCA to the MAOI is far more dangerous than adding the MAOI to the TCA. 2) Clomipramine when combined with an MAOI (particularly tranylcypromine) is far more likely to produce serotonergic syndromes (hyperpyrexic reactions) than are other TCAs. This combination is to be avoided. Lader, in the United Kingdom, has recommended that when switching between an MAOI and clomipramine in either direction, a 4-week interval should be observed (personal communication 1988). 3) Amitriptyline and trimipramine are believed to be the TCAs that "mix best" with an MAOI, i.e., produce less in the way of hypertensive crises. This is largely unproven, although suggestive data do exist. 4) Phenelzine and isocarboxazid appear less problematic than does tranylcypromine, which may have an amphetamine-like action.

MAOI-Trazodone Combinations

Trazodone has been added successfully to MAOIs to reduce insomnia (Nierenberg and Keck 1989). Generally, clinicians should begin at 50–100 mg of trazodone at bedtime, with increases of 50 mg/day every few days to 200 mg at bedtime. In a few patients, myoclonic jerks suggestive of increased serotonergic activity have been reported; however, these reactions have generally been mild and have abated on reduction or discontinuation of trazodone. One Boston clinician noted relief of MAOI-induced impotence in two patients when trazodone was added. The lack of marked serotonergic syndromes with this combination may reflect trazodone's effects on blocking types 1 and 2 serotonin receptors and its weak serotonin reuptake blocking properties.

Trazodone has been combined in very high doses (e.g., 450 mg/day) with MAOIs to treat patients with obsessive-compulsive disorder (see Chapter 6, Baxter et al. 1987). We recommend that clinicians treat obsessive-compulsive patients with other agents before considering this combination.

MAOI-FLUOXETINE COMBINATIONS

MAOI-fluoxetine combinations are potentially as dangerous as those involving MAOIs and clomipramine. Both fluoxetine and clomipramine are potent serotonin reuptake blockers and when used in combination with MAOIs may precipitate serotonergic syndromes characterized by hyperpyrexia, coma, and even death. Treatment of such reactions is supportive; no antidote is known. Early after its release, a few patients who had been on fluoxetine were rapidly shifted to MAOIs and died suddenly, which may have been due to an untoward drug-drug interaction. Because of fluoxetine's long half-life, the manufacturer has recommended waiting 5 weeks before starting MAOIs after fluoxetine is discontinued.

COMBINATIONS OF FLUOXETINE AND OTHER ANTIDEPRESSANTS

Fluoxetine can be combined with TCAs or trazodone to augment antidepressant responses. In animal models, the combination of fluoxetine with desipramine produced marked and rapid downregulation of postsynaptic beta-receptors (Baron et al. 1988), suggesting that the combination should be effective. One recent report suggests this is the case (Weilburg et al. 1989); however, dosing of the TCA must be done very conservatively because fluoxetine will slow the hepatic degradation of TCAs, resulting in potential elevation of TCA levels and increased side effects (Aranow et al. 1989; Bell and Cole 1988). If a tricyclic is added in patients already being treated with fluoxetine, initiation of the TCA should be at low doses: 10 mg of nortriptyline or 25 mg of imipramine with a further increase of 10–25 mg after 3 days. Plasma levels of the TCA should be monitored closely. When fluoxetine is added to the TCA, we recommend first gradually reducing the TCA to 30 mg of nortriptyline or 50–75 mg of imipramine. TCA levels should be obtained before and after dosage reduction as well as after starting fluoxetine (see above).

Trazodone is often safe and useful as a hypnotic in patients with insomnia on fluoxetine. In the course of such use, we found patients whose depressions cleared nicely after trazodone was added to fluoxetine. The trazodone dose needed is between 50 and 300 mg given at bedtime. Adding trazodone is very helpful in perhaps one-third of the patients who have failed to respond to fluoxetine within 4–6 weeks.

TCA–Sedative-Hypnotic Combinations

Not infrequently, depressed patients will require the addition of a sedative-hypnotic to an antidepressant agent. In the case of tricyclics, it is most prudent to use a benzodiazepine, since it will not appreciably alter the pharmacokinetics of the antidepressant. Barbiturates and to some extent chloral hydrate will induce microsomal breakdown of tricyclics in the liver, resulting in lower TCA plasma levels. The prolonged use of these drugs in combination with TCAs should thus be avoided whenever possible. Obviously the use of any hypnotic with another psychotropic also requires monitoring for untoward sedation or central nervous system depression.

Lithium-Anticonvulsant Combinations

Lithium may be combined with anticonvulsants—carbamazepine or valproic acid—in the treatment of patients with refractory mania. There are few, if any, prospective data using such combinations; however, there are a number of reports indicating that lithium-carbamazepine combinations are effective in patients who failed to respond to these two agents given separately (see Chapter 5, Lipinski and Pope 1982; McElroy et al. 1987). No particular untoward interactive effects of lithium with these two agents have been reported. Dosing schedules of the lithium and the anticonvulsant components should parallel regimens used for each drug alone.

Bibliography

Aranow RB, Hudson JL, Pope HG, et al: Elevated antidepressant plasma levels after addition of fluoxetine. Am J Psychiatry 146:911–913, 1989

Baron BM, Ogden AM, Seigel BW, et al: Rapid down-regulation of beta-adrenoreceptors by co-administration of desipramine and fluoxetine. Eur J Pharmacol 154:125–134, 1988

Bell IR, Cole JO: Fluoxetine induces elevation of desipramine levels and exacerbation of geriatric nonpsychotic depression (letter). J Clin Psychopharmacol 8:447–448, 1988

de Montigny C, Grunberg F, Mayer A, et al: Lithium induces rapid relief of depression in tricyclic antidepressant drug non-responders. Br J Psychiatry 138:252–255, 1981

de Montigny C, Cournoyer G, Morissette R, et al: Lithium carbonate addition in tricyclic antidepressant-resistant unipolar depression. Arch Gen Psychiatry 40:1327–1334, 1983

Everett HC: The use of bethanechol chloride with tricyclic antidepressants. Am J Psychiatry 132:1202–1206, 1976

Feighner JP, Brauzer B, Gelenberg AJ, et al: A placebo-controlled multicenter trial of limbitrol versus its components (amitriptyline and chlordiazepoxide) in the symptomatic treatment of depressive illness. Psychopharmacology 61:217–225, 1979

Gitlin MJ, Weiner H, Fairbanks L, et al: Failure of T_3 to potentiate tricyclic antidepressant response. J Affective Disord 13:267–272, 1987

Goodwin FK, Prange A, Post R, et al: Potentiation of antidepressant effects by L-triiodothyronine in tricyclic nonresponders. Am J Psychiatry 139:34–38, 1982

Granacher RP, Baldessarini RJ: Physostigmine: its use in acute anticholinergic syndrome with antidepressant and antiparkinson drugs. Arch Gen Psychiatry 23:375–380, 1978

Heninger GR, Charney DS, Sternberg DE: Lithium carbonate augmentation of antidepressant treatment. Arch Gen Psychiatry 40:1335–1342, 1983

Joffe RT, Singer W: Thyroid hormone potentiation of antidepressants. Neuroendocrinology Letters (St. Michael's Hospital) 9:172, 1987

Kline NS, Pare M, Hallstrom C, et al: Amitriptyline protects patients on MAOI's from tyramine reactions. J Clin Psychopharmacol 2:434–435, 1982

Lemberger L, Rowe H, Bosomworth J, et al: The effect of fluoxetine on the pharmacokinetics and psychomotor responses of diazepam. Clin Pharmacol Ther 43:412–419, 1988

Lipinski JF, Pope HG Jr: Possible synergistic action between carbamazepine and lithium carbonate in the treatment of three acutely manic patients. Am J Psychiatry 139:948–949, 1982

McElroy SL, Pope HG Jr (eds): Use of Anticonvulsants in Psychiatry: Recent Advances. Clifton, NJ, Oxford Health Care, 1988

Nierenberg AA, Keck PE: Management of monoamine oxidase inhibitor–associated insomnia with trazodone. J Clin Psychopharmacol 9:45–54, 1989

Nierenberg AA, Price CH, Charney DS, et al: After lithium augmentation: a retrospective follow-up of patients with antidepressant-refractory depression. J Affective Disord 18:67–175, 1990

Pare CMB, Kline N, Hallstrom C, et al: Will amitriptyline prevent the "cheese" reaction of monoamine oxidase inhibitors? Lancet 2:183–186, 1982

Pope HG Jr, McElroy SL, Nixon RA: Possible synergism between fluoxetine and lithium in refractory depression. Am J Psychiatry 145:1292–1294, 1988

Price LH, Conwell Y, Nelson JC: Lithium augmentation of combined neuroleptic-tricyclic treatment in delusional depression. Am J Psychiatry 140:318–322, 1983

Spiker DG, Weiss JC, Dealy RS: The pharmacological treatment of delusional depression. Am J Psychiatry 142:430–436, 1985

The Upjohn Company: Technical report synopsis: a multicenter study to evaluate the pharmacokinetic and clinical interactions between alprazolam and imipramine. Kalamazoo, MI, The Upjohn Company, 1986

The Upjohn Company: Technical report synopsis: a pharmacokinetic/pharmacodynamic evaluation of the combined administration of alprazolam and fluoxetine. Kalamazoo, MI, The Upjohn Company, 1990

Weilburg JB, Rosenbaum JF, Biederman J, et al: Fluoxetine added to non-MAOI antidepressants converts nonresponders to responders: a preliminary report. J Clin Psychiatry 50:447–449, 1989

Wharton RN, Perel JM, Dayton PG, et al: A potential clinical use for methylphenidate with tricyclic antidepressants. Am J Psychiatry 127:1619–1625, 1971

Wheatley D: Potentiation of amitriptyline by thyroid hormone. Arch Gen Psychiatry 26:229–233, 1972

White K, Simpson G: Combined MAOI-tricyclic antidepressant treatment: a reevaluation. J Clin Psychopharmacol 1:264–282, 1981

Emergency Room Treatment

Psychiatrists see patients in crisis not only in emergency rooms but also (occasionally) in their offices, during home visits, or in medical or nursing home settings. This chapter deals with problems generally within the scope of the psychiatrist functioning without major laboratory or hospital backup.

In emergency situations, psychiatrists are often faced with the diagnosis and treatment of patients presenting with psychiatric symptoms of sudden or presumed recent onset. Phenomenologically, these can be crudely subdivided into

1. Acute psychotic reactions, usually with overt thought disorder, paranoid ideation, and/or hallucinations and marked fear or anger
2. Delirium presenting with disorientation and confusion with or without psychotic symptoms
3. Severe anxiety without psychotic symptoms but often with physical symptoms
4. Anger and belligerent behavior with or without signs of alcohol or other intoxication

10

5. Depression with suicidal ideation with or without a recent suicide attempt
6. Psychogenic stupor

In some of these situations a history can be obtained either from the patient or from friends or relatives. Sometimes the patient may have been carrying enough identification so that friends or relatives can be rapidly contacted. In the worst situation, the psychiatrist will have little to go on besides the patient's behavior and a brief physical examination. When the patient is severely disturbed, obtunded, or confused, can give no history, and has no diagnostic stigmata (e.g., needle tracks, obvious atropine-like toxic signs), hospitalization without specific drug treatment is indicated, or at least medical evaluation with toxic screens, electrocardiogram, etc., in a competent medical emergency facility.

It is necessary to stress the importance of trying to ascertain which drugs the patient has been taking or may have been taking before beginning pharmacotherapy of emergency psychiatric patients. Deaths have occurred when a tricyclic antidepressant or meperidine was given to patients on monoamine oxidase inhibitors. Adding sedative drugs in a patient already intoxicated on alcohol or other sedative drugs is unwise. Adding a neuroleptic to a patient with possible neuroleptic malignant syndrome is obviously contraindicated. Similarly, drugs must be carefully chosen if a tricyclic overdose may have affected cardiac function. In short, when the patient may be on preexisting medication or may have overdosed on an unknown drug it is better to avoid medication until the situation can be clarified.

ACUTE PSYCHOTIC REACTIONS

Psychotic symptoms can be caused by drugs. These should be ruled out by history, physical examination, and urine and/or blood tests for drugs of abuse, wherever possible.

Hallucinogens

Usually lysergic acid diethylamide (LSD) or mescaline or related drugs cause visual illusions and distortions of body image, sometimes with panic, grandiose ideas, or suicidal drive, but patients usually have some knowledge of which drug has been ingested. Even in such a case, potential problems exist because "street drugs" may contain various intended and unintended substances, e.g., mescaline tablets may well contain phencyclidine (PCP) or LSD. Time and a calm, supportive environment enable most such patients to be "talked down." A sedative drug (e.g., 2 mg of lorazepam, or enough to produce sleep) will give time for the hallucinogen to wear off. Antipsychotics have also been used, but are probably not necessary. There are no characteristic physical stigmata of hallucinogenic intoxication. Very large doses of marijuana or hashish can sometimes produce similar states.

Amphetamines

High doses (over 50 mg) of *d*-amphetamine or equivalent doses of related drugs, including methamphetamine, cocaine, and phenylpropanolamine, can produce excited, paranoid psychotic states, usually with a clear sensorium but rarely with delirium. Signs of sympathetic overactivity are less common than would be expected. Patients on prolonged high doses of stimulants can show stereotyped behavior such as picking at spots on the skin, lip biting, or teeth grinding. These states tend to respond to dopamine blocking drugs such as haloperidol. The dose required is a function of the degree of excitement, but 5 mg po or im could be used as an initial dose in disturbed but not wildly excited patients. Hospital admission is generally necessary. Amphetamine psychosis can be treated as though it were a real schizophreniform psychosis (see Chapter 4). Some patients clear in hours or days; others go on to a schizophrenic course of, at best, slow improvement despite adequate medication.

Phencyclidine

PCP can not only produce behavior that mimics paranoid schizophrenia or manic states but can also produce even more bizarre, violent behavior than amphetamines or LSD. There is sometimes muscle tension, tachycardia, hypertension, drooling, horizontal and vertical nystagmus, analgesia, or loss of proprioception with ataxia. Because PCP is best excreted only in acid urine, urine tests can be negative while blood tests are positive; both should be done. PCP psychosis is worsened by environmental stimulation. A benzodiazepine (e.g., 1 or 2 mg of lorazepam po or im) probably is better as emergency medication than a neuroleptic. Patients with severe reactions or symptoms not rapidly abating should be hospitalized.

Anticholinergics

A variety of drugs, including atropine, trihexyphenidyl, and over-the-counter medications containing scopolamine, can induce delirium with psychotic symptoms. Dry, hot, flushed skin, dry mouth, dilated pupils, and tachycardia usually accompany these symptoms. Supportive treatment is indicated, with medical hospitalization.

Physostigmine *will* reverse the symptoms, but only briefly; it can evoke seizures and other adverse effects on its own and should not be used by clinicians who are inexperienced in its use (see Chapter 9).

Alcohol or Sedative Intoxication

Ataxia, slurred speech, confusion, and excitement with belligerent paranoid ideation can be confused with schizophreniform psychosis, but alcohol on the breath or a history of sedative ingestion will often clarify the diagnosis. In chronic alcoholic patients, visual and auditory hallucinosis can complicate the picture.

A differential diagnosis should be made in patients already intoxicated with sedatives to avoid giving additional sedative drugs such as lorazepam or amobarbital.

If tranquilization is needed, an antipsychotic, such as chlorpromazine (25–50 mg by mouth) or haloperidol (5 mg parenterally), is a better choice.

Sedative Withdrawal and Delirium Tremens

Delirium with agitation, tremor, disorientation, hallucinosis, confusion, tachycardia, and hypotension occurs in patients undergoing withdrawal from physical dependence on alcohol, barbiturates, or benzodiazepines. In this instance sedative drugs are needed. When in doubt, 25 mg of chlordiazepoxide could be given stat orally. (See Chapter 11 for details of the treatment of sedative dependence.)

Mixed Psychotic Reactions

With any psychotic reaction presumptively due to illicit or licit drug toxicity, a variety of complicated clinical pictures can and do occur. Illicit drug users often take several kinds of drugs and alcohol simultaneously. Schizophrenic patients abuse drugs and/or become intoxicated on alcohol, and acute drug-induced psychosis can sometimes persist and blend into a picture indistinguishable from schizophrenia that can continue for days or weeks. The pharmacotherapeutic problem is to choose between acute dosages of an antipsychotic versus a benzodiazepine versus watchful waiting while checking for illicit drugs in urine or blood, evaluating possible medical causes, and obtaining a recent history from friends or relatives. A modest oral benzodiazepine dose (e.g., 2 mg of lorazepam, 10 mg of diazepam, or 25 mg of chlordiazepoxide) may be the most conservative option when the diagnosis is in doubt and the patient is very agitated. For parenteral use, lorazepam (1 or 2 mg) is more rapidly and reliably absorbed than are the other parenteral benzodiazepines. Benzodiazepines should not be used in patients who appear already intoxicated on alcohol or sedative drugs.

Schizophrenic, Schizophreniform, or Manic Psychosis

When the likelihood of a drug-induced psychosis is low and the patient is manifestly acutely psychotic—paranoid, disorganized, hallucinated, agitated, belligerent, etc.—some experts recommend rapid neuroleptization (e.g., 10 mg of haloperidol im every 30–60 minutes for up to 4 hours, stopping when the patient becomes calm). There is no real evidence that that much is required. Often oral haloperidol will be taken without objection by the patient; in that case, liquid medication is preferred, since ingestion can be ensured. Whether given by mouth or injection, a single 10-mg dose of haloperidol may well suffice, followed by 5 mg after 2 hours if the patient is still agitated. Other parenteral antipsychotics (e.g., 20 mg of thiothixene, 50 mg of chlorpromazine, 25 mg of loxapine) are probably as effective, although chlorpromazine is more sedative and more likely to cause hypotension. An antiparkinsonian drug (e.g., 2 mg of biperiden) should usually be given at the same time as the neuroleptic to help avert dystonia.

In very severe psychotic excitements, 5 mg im of droperidol will produce sedation and often control excitement within a few minutes. This drug is FDA approved only for "use" in anesthesia but has been used in some psychiatric emergency settings. The available literature strongly supports the value of droperidol in acute emergencies. Rapid sedative control is usually achieved. A few emergency rooms use it heavily. At McLean Hospital, it is used as a backup medication in disturbed patients who do not respond to lorazepam or haloperidol. It is often but not always helpful in tranquilizing very psychotic patients. Lorazepam, 1–2 mg im or iv, will also produce marked sedation on occasion, but intravenous medication should only be used where airway and resuscitation equipment is at hand.

When a psychotic patient can give some history and has a preference among available antipsychotic drugs, or when relatives or past medical records provide relevant information, the "best" past drug for the particular patient should be used.

Delirium

Delirium in medically ill patients seen in emergency rooms should be treated only very cautiously with psychoactive drugs while the underlying medical problem is being diagnosed and treated, preferably after hospital admission.

SEVERE ANXIETY

Patients can present with panic, with severe fear and anxiety, and with multiple somatic symptoms. If medical illness can be rapidly ruled out or the patient has a known history of psychogenic panic attacks, oral diazepam is probably the treatment of choice because of its rapid onset of action after oral administration and its lack of prolonged sedation. Either 5- or 10-mg dosages can be tried, depending on the severity of the anxiety and the patient's past responses to sedatives. Antidepressant drugs are indicated in the longer-term treatment of panic disorders but are slow in onset and of no immediate value in a patient experiencing severe anxiety at the time the first dose is given. Diazepam is probably also the drug of choice in anxiety induced by recent severe stress if the stressful situation has passed. One could argue that alprazolam could be preferred in panic disorder patients presenting in a panic since the drug can both ameliorate the present panic and be continued as a maintenance treatment. It seems better, however, to defer that clinical decision until the acute panic is past (see Chapter 6).

Some experts prefer low-dose antipsychotic drugs in patients with borderline or other personality disorders presenting with an acute crisis, but we know of no evidence favoring an antipsychotic over a benzodiazepine in the emergency room situation. If the patient has a past history of sedative abuse, perhaps 25 mg of chlorpromazine could be tried as a sedative antipsychotic *if* the patient is not currently dependent on sedative drugs. Chlorpromazine's sedation is likely to persist for many hours, longer than is usually desired. If the patient is currently dependent on sedative drugs, consideration must be given to the problem of withdrawal reactions if they are stopped. Buspirone is now available for use in anxiety but is not generally helpful in reducing acute symptoms as a single dose.

Angry Belligerence

In nonpsychotic patients presenting in emergency rooms with angry tantrums, as well as similar patients with severe anxiety that seems to be based on family fights or other interpersonal crises, supportive listening, reassurance, and the elixir of time will often enable the patient to gradually become calm and reasonable without specific medication. Sedative- or alcohol-related angry intoxication will also often pass gradually with time, talk, and external limit setting. If the hostility is severe or persistent, an antipsychotic (perhaps haloperidol 2 mg po or im) can be tried to calm the patient and, hopefully, reduce anger, but no data are available on this use. Benzodiazepine sedatives can sometimes decrease controls and leave the patient more excited and disinhibited.

Depression

Suicidally depressed patients brought to an emergency room after suicide threats or nonharmful attempts present a real challenge to clinical judgment. The conservative course is to admit such patients to a secure inpatient unit. Occasionally, this may seem unwise or impractical. If the clinician can make a relationship with and personally follow the patient—and if friends or relatives can reliably supervise the patient until the next appointment—antidepressant medication can be begun. No antidepressant works fast enough to be dramatically useful in such situations. Trazodone, fluoxetine, bupropion, and alprazolam have the advantage of being relatively safe if taken in overdose with suicidal intent. Some clinicians prefer starting the patient on a standard tricyclic, giving the patient only enough pills to last until the next appointment.

PSYCHOGENIC STUPOR

If medical or neurological causes for stupor can be ruled out, hospital admission to a psychiatric ward is generally indicated. If no information on the patient is available, intravenous amobarbital sodium can sometimes enable a history to be obtained by letting the patient talk relatively freely, but this approach requires a clinician experienced in the technique and, again, is best done in an inpatient setting (see Chapter 6). Parenteral lorazepam (2 mg) can be tried with greater safety and may facilitate relaxation and allow the patient to give a history.

EMERGENCY ROOM REFERRALS

Psychiatric patients occasionally are referred to a general hospital emergency room by their psychiatrist after telephone calls or office visits. Definite or possible overdose attempts, unexplained confusional states, or serious drug side effects (such as MAOI-related hypertensive crises or acute dystonia) are reasonable examples of need for referral.

It is important for psychiatrists to remember that emergency room physicians may know less about the pharmacological effects of psychiatric drugs than they do, despite the natural hope that the emergency room doctor will be all-knowing and highly resourceful. It is therefore worthwhile to call the emergency room before the patient gets there and/or after the patient has been initially evaluated to ensure that no major gaps in knowledge exist. Many physicians have never heard that meperidine can be fatal when added to an MAOI. Some do not know that tricyclic antidepressants have quinidine-like effects on cardiac conduction and might give quinidine to treat an arrhythmia resulting from tricyclic overdose. Although PDR states that hypertensive crises should be treated with Regitine (phentolamine) intravenously, the busy emergency room doctor may not know this and may not read PDR. In emergency rooms it is not uncommon to have a patient with a severe headache due to a hypertensive crisis be ignored (i.e., made to wait) until the headache has passed on its own.

If a patient is sick enough to be admitted to a hospital and the psychiatrist knows of a history of benzodiazepine use, the psychiatrist should encourage the hospital staff to be concerned about withdrawal symptoms such as seizures or delirium. Also, the emergency physician may be reassured to know that overdoses of fluoxetine, trazodone, or bupropion are likely to be relatively benign. In our experience, emergency room staff seem interested and appreciative when the responsible psychiatrist calls and provides both clinical and psychopharmacological input.

Bibliography

Bazire S: MAOIs and narcotic analgesics (letter to the editor). Br J Psychiatry 151:701–710, 1987

Browne B, Lintner S: Monoamine oxidase inhibitors and narcotic analgesics: a critical review of the implications for treatment. Br J Psychiatry 151:210–212, 1987

Cole J: Drugs and seclusion and restraint. McLean Hospital Journal 10:37–53, 1985

Crome P: Antidepressant overdosage. Drugs 23:431–461, 1982

Dubin W, Stolberg R: Emergency Psychiatry for the House Officer. New York, SP Medical & Scientific Books, 1981

Goldberg RJ, Dubin WR, Fogel BS: Behavioral emergencies: assessment and psychopharmacologic management. Clin Neuropharmacol 12:233–248, 1989

Hillard JR (ed): Manual of Clinical Emergency Psychiatry. Washington, DC, American Psychiatric Press, 1990

Hyman S (ed): Manual of Psychiatric Emergencies. Boston, MA, Little, Brown, 1984

Monoamine oxidase inhibitors and anesthesia: an update. International Drug Therapy Newsletter 24:13–14, 1989

Shader R (ed): Manual of Psychiatric Therapeutics. Boston, MA, Little, Brown, 1975 [See Chapters 7, 11, 15, and 20]

Pharmacotherapy of Chemical Dependence

Drug therapies for patients with substance use disorders are sometimes necessary or useful but are rarely sufficient to cure the disorder. The exception is the occasional situation in which illicit drugs are overused by a patient with a major depression to reduce psychic pain or by a patient with mania manifested as overactivity and uncontrolled hedonism. In these situations, appropriate drug therapy for the underlying major psychiatric condition can be very helpful. Unfortunately, some patients with clear syndromes (e.g., depression, bipolar disorder, or schizophrenia) continue to abuse illicit drugs even when in full or partial remission.

There are, however, specific drug therapies for some aspects of chemical dependence. Medications are useful to ameliorate withdrawal symptoms caused by physical dependence on sedative or opiate drugs. Methadone, as maintenance therapy, is a longer-acting, more manageable, less dangerous drug than heroin and can be given indefinitely in an attempt to replace heroin. Naltrexone, an opiate antagonist, can also be given indefinitely to prevent the patient from obtaining

11

euphoria from heroin. Disulfiram (Antabuse) is used in chronic alcoholism to ensure that patients will become unpleasantly sick if they consume alcohol. Serotonin reuptake inhibitors and other serotonergic drugs (e.g., fluoxetine, buspirone) may also have some ability to decrease alcohol intake. Desipramine may be able to reduce cocaine craving during rehabilitation programs.

Some classes of illicit drugs, of course, require no specific drug therapies because they do not cause any serious degree of physical dependence. These include marijuana and the hallucinogens (e.g., lysergic acid diethylamide [LSD], mescaline). Such drugs can be abruptly discontinued, even in heavy and frequent users. Drug dependence syndromes for which drug therapies are sometimes or regularly useful involve stimulants, opiates, sedative-hypnotics, and alcohol.

STIMULANTS

When a patient who is dependent on stimulants is hospitalized, stimulant administration should be stopped abruptly. No tapered withdrawal is necessary.

Patients who have been taking stimulants in large amounts (e.g., over 50 mg of *d*-amphetamine or several doses of cocaine a day) will often have a withdrawal syndrome consisting of depression, fatigue, hyperphagia, and hypersomnia. In unstable individuals this rebound depression could reach serious clinical proportions for a few days and may persist for weeks, usually in less severe form. There have been positive studies of the use of desipramine as a treatment for cocaine abuse, but not for treatment of stimulant abuse. It is not entirely clear whether desipramine, given to a patient coming off a stimulant, is serving as a replacement for the abused stimulant or as a treatment for postwithdrawal depression.

The issue of "abuse" is a problem with medically prescribable stimulants. If the patient has a clinical depression that responds uniquely to stimulants or a clear adult attention-deficit hyperactivity disorder and takes moderate doses in a stable manner to produce socially responsible functioning, perhaps stimulant use may be therapeutically helpful and worth reconsidering if alternative pharmacotherapies fail. If the patient takes stimulants in large doses to get "high" for euphoriant purposes or pushes dosage to the point that paranoia or other serious symptoms develop, then prescribing stimulants is obviously contraindicated. It is not yet clear whether newer, presumptively dopaminergic antidepressants such as bupropion will be more or less useful than desipramine as a maintenance treatment in stimulant users or abusers (see Chapters 3 and 8).

Cocaine abuse is certainly a much more extensive and serious problem than abuse of the older stimulants. Gawin and Kleber have done the most cogent work on the phenomenology and drug therapy of cocaine abuse. Cocaine is usually used in binges of a few hours to a week. When the patient stops, or "crashes," craving may persist for a few hours, but for the next 3–5 days the patient is fatigued, depressed, and eventually sleepy, with increased appetite. The risk of relapse is low during this stage, called Phase 1 by Gawin and Kleber. Over the next 1–10 weeks, the patient progresses from feeling euthymic with mild cocaine craving to a state of high craving with anhedonia, anergia, and dysphoria. If the patient gets through this stage, called Phase 2, then craving becomes only occasional, triggered by conditioned cues.

Several drugs and dopamine agonists such as bromocriptine, amantadine, and L-dopa have been tried in Phase 1, with little obvious efficacy in controlled trials.

Desipramine has been shown to be somewhat effective in reducing dysphoria and craving in Phase 2 (60% abstinence in desipramine patients during the third to sixth week versus 17% abstinence on placebo). The dropout rate was high during the first 2 weeks of the trial before desipramine began to work (Gawin et al. 1989a). Lithium, tried in the same study, had little effect. The problem here is getting an earlier effect from an antidepressant or keeping patients in a controlled environment until desipramine begins to have a noticeable effect on mood and craving. Other antidepressants might do as well, but desipramine was chosen because of its predominant noradrenergic effects and its relatively good side-effect profile. Bupropion, as a putative dopaminergic drug, might be worth trying but has not, to our knowledge, been studied in cocaine-abstinence states.

Buprenorphine, a mixed opiate agonist-antagonist, suppresses cocaine self-administration in monkeys and also decreases substantially the proportion of cocaine-positive urine samples in opiate addicts maintained on it (Kosten et al. 1989). It has not been studied in cocaine addicts to any useful extent. Buprenorphine might be useful in Gawin and Kleber's Phase 1 and Phase 2.

In another approach, the dopamine-blocking neuroleptic flupentixol, which had some probable efficacy in depression in European trials, was given to cocaine addicts in the Bahamas by Gawin et al. (1989b) with promising results. The depot preparation was used. The theoretical basis for this use was that low concentrations of flupentixol might differentially block dopamine autoreceptors, causing increased postsynaptic dopaminergic activity. Flupentixol is available in Canada but is not likely to be available in the United States for some years, if ever. It is possible that low-dose fluphenazine decanoate might have the same effect. This has never been tried.

For the more prolonged Phase 3, which begins after 6 weeks of abstinence and can last for months or years, there is no evidence that desipramine is (or is not) of value. No drug treatment for this prolonged phase has been studied.

Opiates

Detoxification

Abstinence symptoms can begin as early as 6 hours after the last dose of heroin or other short-acting opiates. Withdrawal symptoms include anxiety, insomnia, yawning, sweating, and rhinorrhea, followed by dilated pupils, tremor, gooseflesh, chills, anorexia, and muscle cramps. About a day after the last dose, pulse, blood pressure, respiration, and temperature may all increase, and diarrhea, nausea, and vomiting can occur. The syndrome, untreated, peaks at 2–3 days and resolves within about 10 days, although mild variable complaints may persist for weeks.

Because a great deal of "street" heroin is so weak, some supposed addicts may not have developed true physical dependence. Also, both street and medical opiate users with or without real physical dependence often consciously or unconsciously exaggerate their withdrawal distress in an effort to obtain more opiate medication from the physician. For these reasons the drug treatment of the withdrawal syndrome should be based on objective signs of opiate withdrawal, not on subjective complaints. These are listed in Table 11-1.

Methadone, a long-acting opiate, is used to treat withdrawal because of its superior pharmacokinetics (a long half-life). A short-acting drug like morphine would have to be given every few hours to block withdrawal, whereas methadone accomplishes this when given only twice a day.

The initial methadone dose should be 10 mg orally, in liquid or crushed tablet form so as to blind the patient to that dosage and subsequent dosages during detoxification. The patient should be evaluated every 4 hours, and an additional 10 mg of methadone should be administered if at least two of the four criteria in Table 11-1 are met. Unless the patient is being withdrawn from high-dose methadone maintenance therapy, no more than 40 mg of methadone should be required in the first 24 hours.

The total dosage of methadone given in the first 24 hours should be considered the stabilization dose. This dose is then given the next day in two divided doses (e.g., 15 mg at 8:00 A.M. and 8:00 P.M.) in crushed or liquid form and should be consumed under direct observation of a staff member to

Table 11-1.   Objective opiate withdrawal signs

1. Pulse 10 beats per minute or more over baseline or over 90 if no history of tachycardia and baseline unknown (baseline: vital-sign values 1 hour after receiving 10 mg of methadone)
2. Systolic blood pressure 10 mmHg or more above baseline or over 160/95 in nonhypertensive patients
3. Dilated pupils
4. Gooseflesh, sweating, rhinorrhea, or lacrimation

avoid illicit diversion. The stabilization dose should then be reduced by 5 mg a day until the patient is completely withdrawn.

A patient who is physically dependent on sedative drugs and opiates should be maintained on the stabilization methadone dose without tapering until completely withdrawn from the sedative drug.

An alternative pharmacologic approach to the management of opiate withdrawal has been used for the last few years in some centers. This involves the use of the nonopiate antihypertensive drug clonidine, which has mixed noradrenergic effects. It can suppress both objective and subjective symptoms of opiate withdrawal. In beginning clonidine treatment, the method of Kleber and Kosten is worth following. An initial dose of 0.1 mg of clonidine should be given to assess the patient's tolerance for this approach. Hypotension, dizziness, sedation, and dry mouth are common adverse effects. If the initial dose is tolerated well by the patient, total daily doses of 0.1–0.2 mg every 8 hours can be given during the early phases of opiate dose tapering with increases to as high as 0.2–0.4 mg every 8 hours after 2–3 days. Blood pressure should be checked before each dose, and the dose should not be given if the blood pressure is less than 85/55. Amelioration of withdrawal symptoms reaches a peak at 2 or 3 hours after each dose. Muscle aches, irritability, and insomnia are not well suppressed by clonidine.

In one inpatient study of the use of clonidine in the detoxification of patients coming off maintenance methadone, an average dose of about 1.0 mg of clonidine a day was required for the first 8 days off methadone. In a study using clonidine in outpatient detoxification, the medication was begun at 0.1 mg every 4–6 hours as needed and increased to 0.2 mg every 4–6 hours with a maximum of 1.2 mg a day (average maximum dose was 0.8 mg). Some variation of these dosing strategies could be used if a methadone detoxification program is to be avoided. Physicians interested in using this approach should read the Kosten et al. (1989) article carefully or consult with a local program where this approach is being actively used. Clonidine (Catapres) is available in 0.1-, 0.2-, and 0.3-mg tablets.

Maintenance

For many years, methadone maintenance has been available in major urban areas in specially licensed clinics as a replacement therapy for heroin or other illicit opiates for confirmed addicts who have failed to stay drug free after detoxification. The dose adjustment varies from program to program; doses as high as 80 mg a day are used in some clinics. Patients usually take the drug once a day at the clinic under direct supervision and have their urine samples checked for other illicit drug use. If the patient is drug free and doing generally well, "take homes" are often allowed so that the patient only takes the methadone dose at the clinic every other day. The drug is often dispensed in Tang to avoid intravenous misuse of the alternate-day dose taken at home. Although this regimen would seem to provide a popular and useful alternative for confirmed opiate addicts, patients often drop out of methadone maintenance programs after weeks or months of participation.

LAAM (L-alpha-acetyl-methadone) is even longer acting than methadone and would be effective even if administered only three times a week, eliminating the complications of daily clinic visits and the diversion of "take homes." But, despite extensive study, LAAM is not yet approved for prescription use.

Either methadone or LAAM is intended to avert withdrawal symptoms and to abolish craving for opiates in heroin addicts. It is also supposed to provide so high a level of tolerance to opiates that self-administration of street heroin or other illicit morphine-like drugs will no longer elicit euphoria. Maintenance methadone is stabilizing for some opiate addicts but does not completely suppress drug-seeking behavior even for heroin; patients in methadone programs often continue to get in trouble with other drugs of abuse, especially alcohol and cocaine. Maintenance therapy, even coupled with good support programs, cannot solve the multiple problems of many heroin users. Maintenance methadone is a specialized modality in which psychiatrists cannot get involved in the ordinary course of practice.

Consider the plight of the psychiatrist involved in caring for an opiate-dependent patient who is seeking, or claims to be seeking, admission to a detoxification program but has an admission date that is several days off. What can or should the physician do? It is illegal to prescribe opiates to "sustain an addiction." The best procedure is to consult with the detoxification program staff as to what to do. Under unusual circumstances the psychiatrist could provide the patient with a limited supply of propoxyphene (Darvon), a relatively noneuphoriant opiate, to carry the patient until the admission time. However, the psychiatrist must know the patient well and be sure that he or she is not being tricked or manipulated. Clonidine is an even better alternative. In "medical" addicts—patients who are physically dependent on opiates prescribed for pain relief—it is common to continue the prescription until the patient is admitted to a detoxification unit or chronic pain program.

A newer, currently available maintenance treatment is the opiate antagonist naltrexone (Trexan). This is similar to naloxone (Narcan), the opiate antagonist that has long been available to treat opiate overdose, but naltrexone is much longer acting and available in oral form. Either drug could, in theory, be given orally in large daily doses to create a chronic blockade of opiate receptors, which will reliably block (prevent the euphoriant effects of) heroin or other morphine-like drugs. Naloxone is too weak and short acting orally to be usable. Naltrexone is adequate for the purpose, but to date has had less popularity with opiate addicts than even methadone. However, now that it has become available to the clinician, it may perhaps find a useful niche in the long-term maintenance treatment of some opiate addicts, particularly highly motivated physician-addicts. For the moment, however, naltrexone is still a drug to be used mainly in special programs and not by general psychiatrists unless they are asked to take over a patient who has already been stabilized on naltrexone in a specialty program. The usual dose is 50 mg a day.

The most promising maintenance drug therapy for opiate addicts is buprenorphine, a mixed agonist-antagonist currently available in the United States only as a parenteral injection (Buprenex, 0.3 mg). It is available in Europe also in a sublingual lozenge (0.2 mg). The sublingual route is used to avoid excessive drug destruction in the liver, which occurs if the drug is taken as an ordinary pill and swallowed. This sublingual form is said to be the most widely used analgesic in many European countries, where it is in schedule IV. In the United States the parenteral form is in schedule V.

The drug is a good analgesic but so are many other opiates and mixed agonist-antagonists (e.g., pentazocine). However, when buprenorphine was tested for abuse liability in humans by Jasinki et al. (1978) at the Addiction Research Center, it proved to be well tolerated and to elicit no dependence or withdrawal symptoms even after prolonged high-dose administration.

Buprenorphine can substitute for other opiates and can block opiate-induced euphoria. Preliminary testing for periods of several weeks in opiate addicts suggests that the drug is much more acceptable to patients than naltrexone, perhaps because of a mild euphoriant effect. It decreases illicit drug use, as measured by urine screens, as effectively as methadone—not completely but substantially. It may also decrease cocaine use through blocking the euphoria or perhaps by defeating the "speed ball" combination of heroin and cocaine. In the "speed ball," heroin sedation may balance cocaine stimulation. With the heroin effect blocked, cocaine may be too stimulating.

The probable maintenance dose of buprenorphine is likely to be approximately 4 mg a day, but it is too early to be sure.

The development and testing of buprenorphine as a treatment for opiate addiction has been delayed because the U.S. company that manufactures it has been uninterested in such an alternative use.

SEDATIVES AND HYPNOTICS

Detoxification

Over the last 45 years, the problem of sedative addiction (physical and psychic dependence) shifted from almost completely an abuse of short- or intermediate-acting barbiturates (amobarbital, pentobarbital, secobarbital, etc.) to newer hypnotics (glutethimide, methaqualone) and most recently to benzodiazepines (diazepam, alprazolam, and others). All of these agents (and alcohol) produce cross-tolerance—that is, physical withdrawal symptoms in a patient dependent on any one of these drugs can be relieved by an adequate dose of another. The time course of withdrawal symptoms differs with the half-lives of the drugs involved, coming on within 12–16 hours after the last dose of a barbiturate (e.g., amobarbital or alprazolam) and perhaps 2–5 days after the last dose of diazepam.

Early withdrawal symptoms include anxiety, restlessness, agitation, nausea, vomiting, and fatigue. Later, weakness develops, often with abdominal cramps plus tachycardia, postural hypotension, hyperreflexia, and gross resting tremor. Insomnia and nightmares may occur. Peak symptoms, including grand mal seizures in some instances, occur at about 1–3 days after short-acting drugs (amobarbital, lorazepam, alprazolam) and 5–10 days after long-acting drugs (diazepam, clorazepate). Of patients who have seizures, about half will develop delirium with disorientation, anxiety, and visual hallucinations. Even without seizures, patients in benzodiazepine withdrawal may be mildly confused, perceive lights as being too bright and sounds as too loud, get mildly paranoid, and feel depersonalized.

Sedative withdrawal, particularly from barbiturates, can be fatal, and—once it has progressed to delirium—it is not readily reversible. For this reason, withdrawal from sedative dependence should be considered a medical emergency, and patients presenting in withdrawal should be treated as such. Withdrawal syndromes from benzodiazepines may be less severe. In contrast, opiate withdrawal symptoms are rarely life-threatening and always reversible if an opiate is given.

It is probable that regimens could be worked out for using any long-acting sedative such as phenobarbital, chlordiazepoxide, or diazepam to ameliorate withdrawal from sedatives, but we know of no well-developed medication strategy based on this principle. The most commonly recommended regimen uses the short-acting barbiturate pentobarbital (Nembutal) to establish the degree of dependence and then converts the

patient to the longer-acting phenobarbital for the real detoxification phase.

Pentobarbital Tolerance Test

Once the patient is no longer sedated or intoxicated and is
showing early withdrawal symptoms, 200 mg of pentobarbital should be given by mouth and the patient observed 1
hour later for signs of sedative intoxication. If the patient is
asleep at that point, it is likely that no detoxification is
necessary because the patient has almost no tolerance to the
drug. If the patient has nystagmus, slurred speech, ataxia, or
sedation 1 hour after the initial 200-mg dose, he or she has
probably been taking less than the equivalent of 800 mg of
pentobarbital a day. This patient can then be stabilized on
100–200 mg of pentobarbital every 6 hours, depending on
the degree of sedation induced by the initial 200-mg test
dose.

If the patient shows no response to the initial 200-mg test
dose, he or she requires more than 800 mg a day. To
determine the needed dose, the patient should be given 100
mg every 2 hours until he or she *does* show signs of
intoxication (sedation) or until a total dose of 500 mg of
pentobarbital in 6 hours has been given. The total dose given
in the first 6 hours (300–500 mg) is the patient's 6-hour
requirement, and this dose *could* be given every 6 hours and
gradually tapered by 100 mg a day.

However, it is better to calculate the initial 24-hour
requirement (four times the initial 6-hour dose) and convert
it to phenobarbital at 30 mg for each 100 mg of pentobarbital
(e.g., 1,000 mg a day of pentobarbital requires 300 mg a
day of phenobarbital). The daily phenobarbital dose needed
should be divided into thirds and given every 8 hours for the
first 48 hours.

After 2 days, the phenobarbital dose is decreased by 30
mg a day until the patient is totally withdrawn. Obviously,

if the patient appears oversedated on the calculated dose, it could be slightly reduced, or it could be slightly increased in the face of continuing objective signs of withdrawal.

The above program should be used in patients with patterns of *serious* sedative abuse who have been taking doses large enough to lead to frequent sedative intoxication with behavioral consequences (fights, falls, ataxia, job loss, car accidents) or in patients who combine moderate prescribed benzodiazepine doses (e.g., 30 mg a day of diazepam) with excessive alcohol intake.

For the more common psychiatric patient who has probably become physically dependent on prescribed benzodiazepines at *moderate* doses taken for over a year, the benzodiazepine dose can be gradually decreased while the patient is followed as an outpatient, if the patient can tolerate such a program. There are reports that in panic patients who have responded to relatively higher doses—i.e., 6 mg/day—of alprazolam, reduction in dosage at a rate of 0.5 mg every few days to 2.0 mg/day is generally well tolerated. Further reduction below 2.0 mg/day using this rate of discontinuation will cause patients considerable discomfort. At or below 2.0 mg/day, more gradual reductions by 0.25 mg/day every few days are recommended.

A shift from short-acting benzodiazepines, such as lorazepam or alprazolam, to longer-acting ones like clonazepam can be tried if tapering of the shorter-acting drug leads to uncomfortable symptoms. It is not clear whether rapid inpatient withdrawal is required in such patients, but it seems legitimate if outpatient withdrawal is poorly tolerated. It may be that slow withdrawal over weeks produces more discomfort than a systematic rapid inpatient regimen.

Herman et al. (1987) report good results in shifting patients from alprazolam to clonazepam. He substitutes 1 mg of clonazepam abruptly for every 2 mg of alprazolam and allows patients to take extra doses of alprazolam as needed during the first week on clonazepam. Patients stabilized on clonazepam can then be withdrawn more easily from the longer-acting drug. Carbamazepine has also been used to facilitate withdrawal from alprazolam, with mixed results.

The other issue here is that mild benzodiazepine withdrawal symptoms should be looked for more carefully in patients admitted to psychiatric hospitals who have had their prior sedative benzodiazepine medication abruptly stopped. A few patients appear to become quite uncomfortable with typical withdrawal symptoms after discontinuation of doses as low as 5 mg of diazepam or 30 mg of flurazepam a day if the doses have been taken regularly for many years. Withdrawal symptoms in such patients can last for weeks. Physicians may forget that sedative withdrawal may be occurring when a depressed or schizophrenic patient begins to get more agitated and may be painfully surprised and discomfited when the patient suddenly has a grand mal seizure.

ALCOHOL

Ethyl alcohol is a short-acting sedative drug that produces withdrawal syndromes similar to those caused by the barbiturates. The symptoms and signs of withdrawal are as described under sedative detoxification with the caveat that alcoholic patients either may be very slightly dependent physically but in trouble with alcohol for other reasons or they may be malnourished and/or medically quite ill. Because alcoholism programs tend to treat large numbers of patients, they usually opt for a "standard" detoxification program, which is standard for a given institution but may differ substantially from one facility to another. King's County Hospital in Brooklyn used paraldehyde routinely and successfully for many years; other sites have used phenobarbital, diazepam, or even antipsychotics such as perphenazine or prochlorperazine for alcohol detoxification.

McLean Hospital has used chlordiazepoxide in alcohol

detoxification for at least 15 years; it may be a good choice because it has a long half-life and may be less euphoriant than diazepam. Because of the risk of Wernicke's syndrome in alcoholic patients, thiamine, 100 mg po or im, must be given on admission. Fifty milligrams a day is given daily thereafter for a month. Chlordiazepoxide is initiated at a maximum of 200 mg/day for the first 2 days and is reduced by approximately 25% per day to zero, with extra doses im or po as needed if the withdrawal symptoms are not adequately controlled.

An alternative and perhaps simpler approach developed by Sellers et al. (1983) for alcoholic patients in withdrawal is to administer diazepam in 20-mg doses every 1–2 hours until withdrawal symptoms are relieved. Medication is then stopped, and detoxification is reported to proceed comfortably without further drug treatment once this loading dose of a long-acting benzodiazepine has achieved symptom suppression.

Phenytoin (Dilantin) is added in patients with a history of withdrawal seizures or in patients unable to give an adequate history. The very rare patient developing delirium tremens despite this regimen should be transferred to a major medical hospital for treatment.

Outpatient detoxification has been carried out in patients with adequate motivation and an adequate social support system. Here, 25 mg of chlordiazepoxide taken every 4 hours, or less often if not needed, is probably reasonable for the first day with tapering thereafter (see above). In very tremulous patients who have to be handled as outpatients, a 100-mg im dose of chlordiazepoxide may be indicated. Here the drug's slow absorption from the tissues is an asset, rather than the liability it is in other psychiatric conditions where rapid sedation is the desired effect.

As with opiate withdrawal and maintenance treatment, the general psychiatrist will often be well advised to refer patients to specialized alcoholism programs for, at least, the management of detoxification and possible medical or neurological complications.

Maintenance Treatment

Most alcoholism programs rely mainly on Alcoholics Anonymous plus other educational, psychotherapeutic, and psychosocial modalities. Disulfiram (Antabuse) is often prescribed (or recommended). McLean Hospital uses a daily dose of 250 mg for patients weighing over 170 pounds and 125 mg (half a tablet) for patients under that weight. If the disulfiram is taken daily and alcohol is ingested, the following symptoms appear in this general order: flushing, sweating, palpitations, dyspnea, hyperventilation, tachycardia, hypotension, nausea, and vomiting. These events are usually followed by drowsiness and are usually gone after the patient has slept for a period.

Diphenhydramine, 50 mg parenterally, may be helpful in severe disulfiram-alcohol reactions. Hypotension, shock, or arrhythmias are treated symptomatically. Oxygen is useful in respiratory distress. Hypokalemia may occur. Severe reactions require emergency treatment in a medical setting.

Obviously, the willingness to take disulfiram and thereby commit oneself either to stay off alcohol or suffer unpleasant effects if one drinks is a test of motivation to stay dry. It is still, after all these years, not firmly established that the drug is more than a test of motivation or of compliance with therapy. Long-acting injectable or implantable disulfiram preparations have been tested abroad, but these are not available in this country.

Disulfiram can cause side effects such as fatigue, a metallic taste, rarely impotence, even more rarely toxic psychosis, and very rarely a severe, occasionally fatal toxic hepatitis. The last named side effect comes early in treatment, usually within 2–8 weeks after disulfiram is begun, and is the basis for a labeling recommendation that liver function tests be carried out before disulfiram is begun and again after about 2 weeks of treatment.

Metronidazole (Flagyl) has mild disulfiram-like properties and can cause adverse effects when alcohol is taken with it. Studies of the use of metronidazole in alcoholism have been generally negative.

Beyond disulfiram, there is no specific drug therapy for alcoholism, although individual studies have endorsed such diverse drugs as lithium, propranolol, buspirone, fluoxetine, and chlordiazepoxide. However, none of these is well validated as being effective. Use of lithium carbonate is discussed further in Chapter 5.

There is currently much interest in the potential application of serotonin agonists and reuptake blockers in the management and treatment of patients with alcohol abuse or alcoholism. The rationale stems from a number of observations in lower animals. In rats that are genetically bred to preferentially drink alcohol rather than water, alcohol consumption is reduced by the administration of L-tryptophan and serotonin reuptake blockers (e.g., fluoxetine), but not by noradrenergic tricyclic antidepressants (Naranjo and Sellers 1985). In heavy social drinkers, zimelidine—a serotonin reuptake blocker that was once available in Europe—significantly increased the interval between bouts of consumption. However, subjects drank only about 10% less per bout, suggesting this strategy will only be adjunctive at best. It is currently being pursued by several pharmaceutical concerns in the United States. The mechanism may involve increasing satiety rather than acting via classical aversive or reinforcement mechanisms. It also does not appear to involve their nausea-producing effects. Thus, the use of serotonin reuptake blockers in alcoholism may bear similarity to their application in the management of obesity, a strategy also under active study.

Obviously, if a patient has a drug-responsive psychiatric disorder such as major depression in addition to alcoholism, it should be treated appropriately. The treatment of episodic or chronic residual anxiety symptoms after detoxification is a problem. The use of benzodiazepines is usually frowned upon, probably correctly, although a case could be made that chlordiazepoxide could be considered the sedative equivalent of methadone and might be able to be taken at a stable, controlled rate, whereas alcohol, if used to control anxiety, leads to uncontrolled use. Nonabusable alternatives to sedative benzodiazepines in anxious, abstinent alcoholic patients include propranolol, clonidine, hydroxyzine, tricyclic antidepressants, buspirone, and fluoxetine.

Bibliography

Buffum J, Moser C, Smith D: Street drugs and sexual function. Handbook of Sexology 6:462–477, 1988

Charney D, Sternberg D, Kleber H, et al: The clinical use of clonidine in abrupt withdrawal from methadone. Arch Gen Psychiatry 38:1273–1277, 1981

Cole JO, Ryback RS: Pharmacological therapy, in Alcoholism: Interdisciplinary Approaches to an Enduring Problem. Edited by Tarter R, Sugarman AA. Reading, MA, Addison-Wesley, 1976, pp 687–734

Franks P, Harp J, Bell B: Randomized, controlled trial of clonidine for smoking cessation in a primary care setting. JAMA 262:3011–3013, 1989

Gawin F, Ellinwood E: Cocaine and other stimulants: action, abuse and treatment. N Engl J Med 318:1173–1182, 1988

Gawin F, Kleber H, Buck R, et al: Desipramine facilitation of initial cocaine abstinence. Arch Gen Psychiatry 46:117–121, 1989a

Gawin F, Allen D, Humblestone B: Outpatient treatment of "crack" cocaine smoking with flupenthixol decanoate: a preliminary report. Arch Gen Psychiatry 46:322–325, 1989b

Ginzburg HM: Naltrexone: its clinical utility (DHHS Publ No ADM-84–1358). Washington, DC, U.S. Government Printing Office, 1984

Glassman AH, Stetner F, Walsh BT, et al: Heavy smokers, smoking cessation, and clonidine: results of a double-blind, randomized trial. JAMA 259:2863–2866, 1988

Herman JB, Rosenbaum JF, Brotman AW: The alprazolam to clonazepam switch for the treatment of panic disorder. J Clin Psychopharmacol 7:175–178, 1987

Holloway HC, Hales RE, Watanabe HK: Recognition and treatment of acute alcohol withdrawal syndromes. Psychiatr Clin North Am 7:729–743, 1984

Jasinski DR, Pevnick JS, Griffith JD: Human pharmacology and abuse potential of the analgesic buprenorphine. Arch Gen Psychiatry 35:501–516, 1978

Kosten T: Current pharmacotherapies for opioid dependence. Psychopharmacol Bull 26:69–74, 1990

Kosten T, Vileber H: Buprenorphine detoxification from opioid dependence: a pilot study. Life Sci 42:635–641, 1988

Kosten TR, Kleber HD, Morgan C: Role of opioid antagonists in treating intravenous cocaine abuse. Life Sci 44:887–892, 1989

Mason NA: Disulfiram-induced hepatitis: case report and review of the literature. DICP 23:872–875, 1989

Mirin S (ed): Substance Abuse and Psychopathology. Washington, DC, American Psychiatric Press, 1984

Naranjo CA, Sellers EM: Research Advances in New Psychopharmacological Treatments for Alcoholism. New York, Excerpta Medica, 1985

Rosenbaum JF (ed): New uses of clonazepam in psychiatry. J Clin Psychiatry 48:3S–56S, 1987

Sellers T, Naranjo C, Harrison M, et al: Diazepam loading: simplified treatment of alcohol withdrawal. Clin Pharmacol Ther 34:822–826, 1983

Shader R (ed): Manual of Psychiatric Therapeutics. Boston, MA, Little, Brown, 1975 [See Chapters 11–14]

Smith D, Wesson D: Phenobarbital techniques for treatment of barbiturate dependence. Arch Gen Psychiatry 24:56–60, 1971

Sullivan JT, Sellers EM: Treatment of the barbiturate abstinence syndrome. Med J Aust 145:456–458, 1986

Washton A, Resnick R: Clonidine for opiate detoxification: outpatient clinical trial. Am J Psychiatry 137:1121–1122, 1980

Weiss RO, Mirin SM: Intoxication and withdrawal syndromes, in Manual of Psychiatric Emergencies. Edited by Hyman S. Boston, MA, Little, Brown, 1984, pp 217–227

Pharmacotherapy in Special Situations

Most published reports evaluating the efficacy of psychoactive drugs in psychiatric patients carefully select physically healthy, adult but nonelderly patients. Unfortunately, in clinical practice, physicians frequently encounter patients with psychiatric disorders who are also medically ill, pregnant, brain-damaged, elderly, or juveniles, but who are otherwise appropriate candidates for conventional pharmacotherapy. This chapter will address some of these problems.

PREGNANCY

12

Pregnancy, current or planned for the future, poses a complex problem for the psychiatrist and for the psychiatric patient and her fetus. Pregnancy does not protect patients against the occurrence or recurrence or exacerbation of psychiatric conditions. Depression, mania, and schizophrenia may all occur or worsen during pregnancy, although postpartum depression may be more of a problem than depression during pregnancy.

The risks of drug administration during pregnancy include teratogenesis, particularly during the first trimester, and possibly "behavioral teratogenesis." Gross physical malformations are easy to detect and document, and the possibility that drugs given during pregnancy may affect brain function and behavior years later exists, but there is no clear evidence that it actually occurs. Direct toxic effects on the fetus can occur later in pregnancy. Drugs can affect labor and delivery,* with residual effects on the infant's behavior after delivery. Drugs are also usually excreted in the mother's milk during breast-feeding, sometimes in concentrations sufficient to affect the infant. All this puts both doctor and patient in a very unpleasant bind. Ideally, every mother should be totally drug free throughout every pregnancy.

This problem area is illustrated by the case of a markedly manic drug-free patient believed to be in the sixth week of pregnancy who was once admitted to McLean Hospital. She was kept drug free in seclusion, and often in restraint, for a week because the treating psychiatrist was afraid to initiate neuroleptic treatment for fear of harming the fetus. One of us consulted on the case and advised proceeding with haloperidol therapy despite the presumed pregnancy on the grounds that severe hyperactivity and distress were a risk to both patient and fetus, whereas there was no direct evidence that haloperidol or any other neuroleptic leads to any specific birth defect. The physician in charge disagreed. Finally, an ultrasound examination revealed a false pregnancy, and appropriate drug treatment was begun. This case illustrates one kind of clinical dilemma. Thalidomide, with its gross fetal deformities, still haunts all of pharmacotherapy.

As far as we can determine, the only drugs commonly used in psychiatry with proven relationships to specific birth defects are lithium salts and most anticonvulsants. Lithium has been associated with cardiac abnormalities, especially Ebstein's anomaly, and anticonvulsants have been associated with a variety of birth defects, including facial deformity and spina bifida.

Beyond this, there is no clear evidence that any standard psychiatric drug does (or does not) cause birth defects. Congenital abnormalities occur in babies born to mothers who are taking no drugs at all, but there is a general suspicion that any drug *might* be bad for the fetus, and no doctor feels comfortable recommending drug therapy for a female patient who is believed to have recently become pregnant, or who intends to become pregnant. Of course, whenever possible, drug therapy should be avoided in such instances.

Unfortunately, there are some women with severe, even disabling psychiatric disorders who either wish to become pregnant or actually become pregnant, and a choice must be made between treating the patient and avoiding medicating the fetus. If the situation is not a crisis, as in the patient who is on maintenance medication but would like to become pregnant, outside consultation can be obtained from a psychiatrist experienced in working collaboratively with obstetricians or from a dysmorphologist (an expert in birth defects), a type of specialist found in major medical centers. Telephone hot lines providing information on the effects of drugs on the fetus are also available. One of these, the Pregnancy Environmental Hotline (Teratogen Information Service, National Birth Defect Center), is located at the Kennedy Memorial Hospital in Brighton, Massachusetts. Its telephone number is (617) 787–4957. Staff members are willing to accept calls and refer callers to other programs around the country when appropriate. Major reference works in this area are listed in the bibliography of this chapter.

The information from the psychiatrist, dysmorphologist, or telephone hot line will indicate whether there is any solid evidence that a particular drug is teratogenic, but it will not solve the clinician's whole problem. The final decision must be based on the seriousness of the patient's distress and the reasonableness of the desire to have a child. Documented informed consent from the patient and her family (including her husband or her parents, when appropriate) for the treatment plan are necessary whether one decides to leave the patient drug free with the risks of that course, or to continue with a needed medication despite the pregnancy.

If it seems likely that the patient will relapse if taken off her medication or it is unclear how fast pregnancy is likely to occur, one might keep the patient on medication until the first period is missed. It is likely that stopping medication 2 weeks into pregnancy is early enough to avoid malformations. The same reasoning holds for patients who become accidentally pregnant while on psychiatric drugs.

If one can avoid medication for the first 3 months of pregnancy, then the risk of fetal abnormality is much reduced, but other risks can occur. Babies born to mothers who are physically dependent on sedatives or opiates will suffer withdrawal syndromes and will need to be treated postnatally. We have heard a rumor of a baby being born with a dystonic reaction when the mother had been on neuroleptics. Autonomic withdrawal symptoms presumably could occur in the newborn if the mother has been on tricyclic antidepressants (TCAs). One can justify withdrawing medication carefully from pregnant women a few weeks before delivery.

After the baby is born, nursing mothers on medication will probably excrete drug in breast milk. In the absence of data on breast milk concentrations of a specific drug, it is hard to estimate the seriousness of this problem, but generally breast milk concentrations are lower than drug levels in the blood and the total dose ingested by the infant may be quite small. If a reliable laboratory procedure is available for the drug the mother is receiving, the actual drug levels in the mother's milk can be determined. There is a general belief that mothers on psychiatric medications should not nurse their babies.

Another concern is the possibility that drug therapy with a psychoactive drug during pregnancy (or nursing) may somehow affect brain development in the child. There are really no data on which to base this concern or with which to reassure the patient.

As with many risk-benefit situations in medicine, the suffering or psychiatric hospitalization of the mother must be weighed against the often unknown risk to the infant as interpreted by the doctor, the patient, and the patient's family. A local psychiatrist (L. Cohen, M.D.) at Massachusetts General Hospital specializes in psychiatric aspects of pregnancy and childbearing. We have found his consultation and recent reviews helpful in this area (see Bibliography).

CHILDREN AND ADOLESCENTS

Prepubescent children have efficient livers. This generally allows them to metabolize drugs rapidly and enables them to tolerate somewhat higher doses of psychiatric drugs per unit of weight than adults tolerate. After puberty, drug metabolism resembles that seen in young adults. The lesson here, of course, is not that 7-year-olds should be given huge doses of drugs but that they should be started on very small doses. If there is no response, the dose may be gradually increased to adult dosages, adjusted for weight, without fear of unusual toxicity.

On the other hand, there are no studies at all of the long-term consequences of psychiatric drug therapy in childhood on brain function, behavior, or physical health in adult life. The decision to use a drug treatment for a psychiatrically ill child or young adolescent must therefore be based on a clear and urgent clinical need. The psychiatric disorder must pose significant danger to the child's development and well-being and should only be undertaken after considered medical and psychiatric evaluation.

It should be noted that most standard psychiatric drugs have not received FDA approval for "use" in children or even in adolescents, mainly because the necessary studies have not been carried out.

Stimulants

The best studied and best validated drug therapy for psychiatrically ill children is the use of stimulants—d-amphetamine, methylphenidate, and magnesium pemoline (see Chapter 8)—in attention-deficit hyperactivity disorder (ADHD). Caffeine is not effective in this condition. TCAs (e.g., desipramine) in low dosages (10–75 mg a day) may be useful but may act more slowly. Their effects have been said to fade after a few months. Stimulants often show effects in hours; TCAs may take days or weeks. Research on the effects of stimulants on various kinds of behavior suggests that the drug effects are complex. The dose that controls overactivity best may be too high for optimal improvement in learning. The stimulants may cause slight decrease in body growth, perhaps 1–3 cm in height over the entire developmental period, though a recent follow-up study showed no effect of stimulant exposure on adult height. Children on stimulants may show side effects such as anorexia, insomnia, dysphoria, and even tics. On the other hand, some children with ADHD are markedly benefited, generally more in behavior than in academic performance, whereas others are somewhat better and a few are not benefited or even become more agitated. Of the available stimulants, d-amphetamine and methylphenidate are a bit more effective and safer than magnesium pemoline. Magnesium pemoline can cause hepatocellular damage, presumably due to toxic metabolites, in 1–3% of children treated. Monthly tests of liver function are in order if magnesium pemoline is used.

Some children respond better, unpredictably, to one of the three stimulants than to the other two. d-Amphetamine has the advantage of being generally cheaper. Amphetamine, methylphenidate, and methamphetamine are short acting and generally must be given twice a day, on arising and around noon. For school children, a lunchtime dose may pose problems. Pemoline is longer acting, and a single morning dose may be sufficient. Sustained-release preparations of *d*-amphetamine, methylphenidate, and methamphetamine are available, but their usefulness in ADHD children is not well documented. They can certainly be tried if a once-a-day dose is desired or needed. In patients with a good stimulant response, drug holidays every few months to see if the drug is still needed are worth trying. The practice of giving a child with ADHD medication only on school days may have the disadvantage of impairing the child's family and peer relationships as well as impairing learning outside the school situation. Some children continue to benefit from stimulants into adolescence or even adulthood. Dosage may need to be adjusted, up or down, over time as the child grows and matures.

Antipsychotics

In autistic or psychotic children, neuroleptics are often used with some benefit. These conditions in children under age 15 rarely show marked improvement with antipsychotic treatment, although some decrease in overactive, disorganized behavior can occur. There is no evidence that children are any less tolerant of these drugs than are adults, except perhaps for an even higher rate of dystonia early in treatment in adolescents. However, the risk of tardive dyskinesia and the lower likelihood of marked improvement make it necessary that clinicians use these agents cautiously, documenting carefully the clinical effects observed, and periodically assessing the patient off medication to make sure the treatment is really useful as a maintenance therapy. In older adolescents, acute psychotic syndromes begin to resemble those seen in adults and may be treated in the same manner (see Chapter 4). Sedative neuroleptics (e.g., thioridazine and chlorpromazine) may interfere with learning. Of the nonsedative neuroleptics, haloperidol has been best studied in children with autism (pervasive developmental disorder) and has limited efficacy.

Antipsychotics in low dosages (e.g., 0.5–3 mg of haloperidol or 2–10 mg of pimozide a day) can also control the tics of Tourette's disorder; clonidine has also been reported to be helpful in severe cases of this disorder. Clonidine can suppress tics fairly well but may be more effective in Tourette's patients with explosive violent behaviors. Clonidine causes dry mouth, sedation, constipation, and hypotension. Antipsychotics have often been used to control the behavior of angry, impulsive children and adolescents without psychosis. This use is not well validated but most clinicians use low doses of neuroleptics to control angry, violent behavior in child or adolescent inpatients. Some prefer haloperidol in low doses (e.g., 2 mg every hour until the patient is calm), whereas others use more sedative drugs like chlorpromazine in 10- to 50-mg doses three or four times a day. The one well-controlled study (Platt et al. 1984) comparing haloperidol (2–6 mg a day), lithium carbonate, and placebo in hospitalized nonpsychotic aggressive children with conduct disorder showed the two drug regimens to be more effective than placebo on various measures. The nursing staff judged the lithium responders to have done best. Sedation and dystonia were problems in patients on haloperidol. The risks and benefits of this use are unclear. If antipsychotics are used to reduce aggression in children with conduct disorder and actually are effective, the continued use of these potentially harmful drugs to control deviant behavior must be strongly justified. For each particular patient, the drug must make a major and clinically important difference.

The side effects of antipsychotics, including tardive dyskinesia, are essentially same in children as in adults. However, the possibility of cognitive blunting with these drugs may be relatively more of a problem in children. An inert child who is not learning or functioning may be less trouble to others but may develop more normally if medication is reduced or stopped.

When neuroleptics are used in children or adolescents, documented informed consent from the responsible parent or parents is mandatory. Even if the child or adolescent is too young to give informed consent, the risks and benefits of the drug should be explained to the patient, and his or her assent to the treatment should be obtained when possible (see Chapter 1).

Antidepressants

TCAs are effective in the treatment of enuresis at doses of 0.3–1.0 mg/kg of imipramine or equivalent drugs, but behavioral treatments are generally preferred because they are also effective and may have a lower relapse rate. ADHD tends to respond in the same dosage range. It is interesting to note that tricyclics improve enuresis within a few days, whereas response to ADHD or depression takes 1–4 weeks. Monoamine oxidase inhibitors (MAOIs) are also said to be effective in both enuresis and ADHD but their use is not well studied. Bupropion has some documented efficacy in ADHD.

Some children clearly meet conventional adult criteria for major depressive disorder and respond to TCAs. FDA guidelines recommend an upper dosage limit of 2.5 mg/kg for imipramine; however, some studies report dosages up to 5.0 mg/kg as often being necessary for clinical response. Monitoring of cardiac function is wise when tricyclics are used in children, with ECGs being done prior to starting therapy, again when the dosage exceeds 3 mg/kg, and then every 2 weeks if dosage is being increased. Doses over 5 mg/kg should not be used without outside consultation. Significant slowing of cardiac conduction (P-R interval over 0.20, QRS interval over 0.12) may require lowering the dose.

Side effects of antidepressants in children resemble those seen in adults. Blood level monitoring is about as useful as it is in adults. Imipramine is the best studied drug, and positive correlations between blood level and improvement are often found in clinical trials.

Local experience at McLean Hospital suggests that depressive symptoms in adolescents rarely include major appetite changes or early morning awakening. Overly sound and lengthy sleep with dysphoria on awakening are more common. Physical symptoms, fatigue, irritability, anger, and retardation for the first few hours in the day may be present without subjective recognition of depression or sadness. Sex drive is decreased. These adolescents often have a family history of affective disorder. This pattern often responds to TCA therapy, although formal controlled studies have not been done. Panic agoraphobia can occur in adolescents and can be treated with antidepressants.

Given the cardiac problems that can potentially occur with TCAs and the difficulties with diet with MAOIs, the use of the newer heterocyclic antidepressants (fluoxetine, bupropion, and trazodone) deserves cautious trials in depressed children and adolescents. All three are quite safe in overdose. In adjusting dosages for younger children, fluoxetine's forthcoming oral elixir should be useful. Until it arrives, dissolving 20 mg of fluoxetine in apple or cranapple juice and administering 5 mg a day initially seems reasonable. Tablets of trazodone or bupropion can be broken in halves or quarters, but with difficulty. Until a psychiatrist or clinical facility has extensive experience with any of these drugs, assent from the patient and informed consent from the parent should be obtained.

Clomipramine is now available for the treatment of obsessive-compulsive disorder. It has been shown to be effective in children and adolescents with this condition (see Chapter 6 for additional discussion).

Lithium

Adolescents can show a typical bipolar picture that often responds to lithium therapy. Preadolescent children rarely show mania but can show cyclic mood and behavior shifts with periods of impulsivity, social intrusiveness, tantrums, mood lability, and nonpsychotic euphoria with parallel shifts in vegetative symptoms, which sometimes respond to lithium. The side effects of lithium are the same in children as in adults. To date, no one knows the long-term consequences of long-term maintenance lithium treatment begun in childhood or adolescence.

Antianxiety Drugs

Benzodiazepines are sometimes of use for short periods in pavor nocturnus, or sleepwalking. If used for daytime anxiety, they can increase activity and produce or aggravate behavior disorders, particularly in children with ADHD. Severe school phobia is better treated with imipramine, although a single dose of a benzodiazepine may be used occasionally to allay anticipatory anxiety and help a child return to a feared situation for the first time.

Sedative antihistamines are believed to have some antianxiety or hypnotic utility in children for short periods. Prolonged use could lead to anticholinergic side effects and cognitive impairment.

It is worth remembering that newer drugs are rarely studied in children or adolescents prior to marketing, and even the older drugs are often only partially studied in children and adolescents. The place of drug therapy in children and adolescents is still controversial. Drugs should be reserved for clearly distressed or dysfunctional conditions where psychosocial treatments either have failed or are only likely to be of short-term benefit. Drug therapy needs to be carefully monitored and requires close collaboration between the physician, the parents, and often school personnel or other caretakers. Prolonged maintenance drug therapy is sometimes justifiable, but there should be strong clinical evidence of benefit, and trials off medication are often indicated to make sure the drug is still making a useful difference.

GERIATRIC PATIENTS

Elderly psychiatric patients present a variety of potential problems for the psychiatrist considering prescribing psychoactive drugs. The elderly may have decreased ability to metabolize some drugs, although this has been documented only infrequently. They *may* have low serum protein levels, which could lead them to have relatively higher levels of free drug (not bound to protein) at any given blood level; free drug is usually presumed to be more active and more likely to cross the blood-brain barrier. The elderly *may* be more sensitive to peripheral side effects (e.g., hypotension, constipation) than younger patients at the same dose or blood level. They *may* also be more prone to central side effects (e.g., delirium, tremor, tardive dyskinesia). None of these presumptions is well documented except for delirium and tardive dyskinesia, chiefly because no adequate studies have been done.

Probably the elderly have a reduced reserve of both brain function and cardiovascular competence, which leaves them more vulnerable to drug side effects. In addition, the consequences of side effects, such as falls due to orthostatic hypotension, falls due to confusion, or ataxia or decubitus ulcers due to prolonged oversedation, are more likely to be serious in the elderly. The situation is made worse by the higher likelihood of coexisting medical illness and the use of other drugs for these illnesses in the elderly as well as by the lack of any clear criteria for predicting which elderly patients need very low, cautious dosage regimens of psychoactive drugs and which patients will require (and tolerate) rather large dosages to attain adequate treatment response.

For the standard psychiatric conditions such as depression, mania, chronic schizophrenia, generalized anxiety disorder, etc., the only safe and reasonable approach is to begin with very low drug dosages and to increase the dosage cautiously. As an example, 25 mg of imipramine or trimipramine at bedtime is a reasonable starting dose for healthy patients over age 60, and a 10-mg dose is reasonable for patients over age 70 or for patients over age 60 with concurrent medical problems or with evidence of organic dementia. In such patients, dosage increments should occur every 3–7 days, not every day, so that the clinician has a chance to assess side effects before increasing the dose. Other antidepressants, such as trazodone, fluoxetine, bupropion, and MAOIs, and electroconvulsive therapy (ECT) have been used effectively in elderly patients with major depressions.

In recent years there has been an increasing popularity of nortriptyline in the first-line treatment of depression in patients over age 65. Reasons for this preference include a decreased likelihood of orthostatic hypotension, a mild satisfactory hypnotic effect without continuing sedation the next morning, and somewhat fewer anticholinergic side effects. Recent local experience, confirmed by discussions with other geriatric psychiatrists and family practitioners, suggests that fluoxetine has been, generally, a disappointment in hospitalized elderly depressed patients. Fluoxetine does not appear to be as effective as nortriptyline, and its side effects of agitation, insomnia, and daytime sedation are not well tolerated. It does not cause orthostatic hypotension or other cardiac effects. Perhaps much lower doses with the anticipated liquid elixir formulation will be better received.

Trazodone should be a good drug in elderly depressed patients and can be an excellent hypnotic. It should not cause orthostatic hypotension except for a couple of hours after a bedtime dose. However, occasional patients in their 70s and

80s do have daytime hypotension when treated with trazodone.

ECT remains the major treatment for depressed elderly patients when drug therapy fails. It often is very effective. However, some patients with recurring depressions stop responding to ECT after the 3rd–10th course of treatment for unknown reasons.

Although stimulants are occasionally quite helpful in recent-onset depressions in elderly patients with medical problems, they often only induce agitation in treatment-resistant elderly depressed patients.

Another presumption in the treatment of elderly patients is that anticholinergic drugs increase the likelihood of delirium. On this basis, desipramine should be safer than amitriptyline and fluphenazine safer than thioridazine. Our review of the literature on tricyclic use in the elderly suggests, however, that delirium more often occurs in patients on a tricyclic-neuroleptic combination and that this side effect can be transient and relatively easily managed. Again, there are no adequate controlled trials documenting this issue.

If benzodiazepines are to be used as hypnotics or for daytime anxiety, again use the lowest dose (e.g., 2 mg of diazepam or 0.125 mg of triazolam) first to see whether this dose is adequate and to make sure side effects do not occur. There is evidence that benzodiazepine metabolism is slowed in the elderly and a presumption that higher, cumulative blood levels will be associated with behavioral toxicity. Occasionally, elderly (and young adult) patients will complain of excessive morning sedation after slowly metabolized hypnotics like flurazepam, but there is a good deal of individual variability in the extent to which this consequence of slowed metabolism actually causes demonstrable clinical problems.

Lithium excretion is, on the average, slowed in the elderly as a consequence of an age-related decrease in kidney function. Therefore, older patients should be started on low doses— 300 mg a day in patients in their 60s and early 70s and 150 mg a day in patients who are older. Lithium levels and clinical signs of toxicity should be watched for scrupulously. It is our impression that the elderly can slip from therapeutic to toxic blood levels more rapidly and insidiously than young adult patients. On the other hand, lithium can be as effective in some older bipolar patients as it is in younger ones, although some elderly patients with a late onset may have a simultaneous organic disorder that does not respond well to lithium.

In older chronic schizophrenic patients, there is a belief that lower antipsychotic dosages are needed than in younger adult patients. There is, again, no real evidence that this is true, but there is some evidence that the same antipsychotic dose yields blood levels 1.5–2 times higher in elderly than in younger patients. Cautious attempts at gradually tapering dosage are indicated in schizophrenic patients over age 60 who are on maintenance neuroleptic treatment. When such patients have stopped their medication and become acutely psychotic, cautious low-dosage medication (e.g., 0.5–2 mg a day of haloperidol or fluphenazine) should be tried for the first week to see if a clinical response can be obtained without resorting to high dosages. However, if the patient fails to improve and has a history of requiring and tolerating higher neuroleptic dosage, the dose can be gradually raised, again watching for side effects. The use of antiparkinsonian drugs *could* cause delirium, but leaving the patient with dystonia or pseudoparkinsonism is equally undesirable; the clinician is forced to feel his or her way, attempting to maximize benefit and minimize adverse effects. This applies equally to the use of neuroleptics in younger adult patients, but—in the elderly—the problems encountered in attempting to achieve the right balance of medications may be more frequent.

Tardive dyskinesia is statistically more prevalent in elderly patients, especially women, on maintenance neuroleptics, but in chronic schizophrenic patients the dyskinesia usually has already been present for years and is not a contraindication to using neuroleptics to achieve relief of psychotic symptoms. In the rare chronic patient showing new dyskinesia, a trial off neuroleptics is usually indicated. The concurrent presence of both pseudoparkinsonism and dyskinesia in the same patient is more common in the elderly than in other patients.

Elderly Patients With Dementia

Most elderly patients with mild, moderate, or severe dementia have Alzheimer's disease, although some have multi-infarct dementia, a few have both, and some have neither. The best treatment for dementia is to diagnose a treatable, reversible cause such as vitamin deficiency, hypothyroidism, or congestive heart failure and to treat the underlying medical condition. The other confounding diagnosis is pseudodementia secondary to major depression. Some authors believe that depression can, in fact, cause dementia in the elderly, and depression can certainly aggravate mild, preexisting cognitive dysfunction. The evidence is clear that depression should be carefully and thoroughly treated when cognitive impairment and depression coexist.

Antidepressants should also be used in patients with strokes or organic mood lability even if the depressive syndrome is only partially present. The odds favor a substantial improvement over any worsening of organic deficit, although dosage should be started low and raised cautiously. It *is* clear that patients with behavioral deficits due to strokes who show insomnia, weight loss, agitation, and inability to participate in rehabilitative programs can do well on TCAs and presumably on other antidepressants. There are several favorable reports on the use of nortriptyline in post-stroke depression. This strategy was undertaken because nortriptyline is less likely to produce orthostatic blood pressure changes at therapeutic blood levels than are other TCAs (see below). Just because the dysphoria *seems* appropriate to the disability, treatment should not be withheld.

Dementia alone is no indication, to date, for drug therapy. The only drug marketed in the United States for senile symptoms, ergoloid mesylates (Hydergine), does seem to regularly be a bit more effective than placebo in a large number of double-blind, placebo-controlled studies, but the effects are weak, different in different studies, and usually only manifest after 2–3 months, making the marginal utility of this treatment questionable. A variety of drugs have been studied in dementia, including piracetam, vincamine, lecithin, oral physostigmine, etc., but so far none has been shown to be regularly and safely useful.

Since 1986 there has been a flurry of interest in tetrahydroaminoacridine (THA), an old Australian drug used there to reverse drug-induced coma. It is a central cholinesterase inhibitor that should act by raising brain acetylcholine levels and increasing cholinergic brain activity. After an initial very positive study published in the *New England Journal of Medicine* (Summers et al. 1986), a controlled multicenter trial of THA in Alzheimer's dementia was initiated by the National Institute on Aging. Unfortunately, THA appears to cause hepatotoxicity in some patients, slowing the progress of the trial. It seems likely that THA will ultimately be neither as effective nor as safe as the original article suggested but probably will be shown to cause statistically significant but modest improvement in memory and/or behavior. Similar studies of physostigmine, a much shorter acting cholinesterase inhibitor, are also in progress, with occasional patients showing modest benefits in memory and performance.

Patients with chronic dementia sometimes show agitation, irascibility, night wandering, paranoid ideation, or hallucinations and become major management problems at home or in psychiatric hospitals or nursing homes. Many of these patients are routinely treated with neuroleptics, often with dubious benefit. A recent review of the few controlled studies in this area suggests that only a third of these patients clearly benefit from low-dose neuroleptics (Cole 1990). In our own experience, thioridazine is not better tolerated than low doses of more potent antipsychotics; all neuroleptics show an unfortunate tendency to cause pseudoparkinsonism and akathisia in the elderly. These, plus the increased risk of tardive dyskinesia and the probably increased risk of organic confusional states when antiparkinsonian drugs are added, make neuroleptics often unsatisfactory drugs in agitated, demented patients. Sometimes they are very helpful, but more often the side effects limit their usefulness. They tend to be overused because clinicians believe they lack other options. Locally we see elderly demented patients on neuroleptics with distressing pseudoparkinsonism and akathisia who appear to be more agitated than they were before the neuroleptic was begun 2 or 3 weeks earlier. Perhaps starting with even lower antipsychotic doses or tapering the dose after initial agitation and/or psychosis is reduced would help avert these distressing consequences of well-intentioned antipsychotic therapy.

Are there other medication options in anxious or agitated demented patients? None have been well studied. Probably some patients would respond to a benzodiazepine, preferably oxazepam because of its simple metabolism and low abuse potential. This drug at least offers hope of an early response when the dose is adjusted properly.

Other drugs have been the subject of individual case reports. Propranolol has been most widely studied but mainly in organic agitation and assaultiveness in nonelderly brain-damaged patients. Some case reports suggest that agitation decreases as soon as the right dose of propranolol is reached, but most studies report improvement after a month on the right dose. In the hospitalized, agitated, restless, irascible demented patient, a month is a long, long time, and propranolol carries the risk of orthostatic hypotension with resulting falls. If it is to be tried in elderly patients, the starting dose should be 10 mg twice a day, increased in increments of 10–20 mg every 2 days to 200 mg a day, stopping at lower doses if hypotension or other side effects occur. Propranolol can cause delirium. Glassman's group has shown that orthostatic hypotension due to TCAs is far worse in cardiac patients on multiple cardiac medications than in medically healthy depressed patients. The same seems likely with propranolol—it probably should not be tried in patients on multiple cardiac or other medications.

There are brief case reports of trazodone and buspirone being helpful in agitated elderly demented patients.

Psychosocial measures may be more useful than drugs in elderly patients with dementia. If neuroleptics are used and the patient's behavior is controlled on them for months, the drug should be tapered and stopped from time to time to make sure it is really helping and to make sure tardive dyskinesia is not being masked by the neuroleptic.

Better studies of more kinds of drug therapy are needed in elderly patients, but in their absence, clinicians have to cautiously try to do their best with available measures.

MENTAL RETARDATION

As with the demented elderly, the institutionalized mentally retarded have been treated routinely for decades with neuroleptics, mainly thioridazine, for a wide range of behavioral disorders. Court decisions have mandated evaluation of such patients off medications, and it now appears that only a fraction of those receiving long-term neuroleptic medication are clinically better on them than off them. The neuroleptic-responsive retarded patients have not been well characterized, but it seems probable that some show psychotic symptoms that would qualify for a diagnosis of schizophrenia.

A general principle in the treatment of mentally retarded patients may be useful as a guideline. Such patients often show aberrant behaviors (disrobing, jumping, poking fingers in eyes, etc.) that can increase dramatically when the patient becomes psychiatrically upset. Counting (monitoring) these target behaviors can be a useful guide to treatment effect in often nonverbal patients. The "real diagnosis" may have to be inferred from changes in vegetative symptoms such as sleep, appetite, and motor activity or family history of psychiatric disorders.

All this gives a trial-and-error quality to the drug therapy of the behaviorally disturbed mentally retarded patient, reinforcing Sovner's practice of monitoring target behaviors or symptoms before and during trials. It may take a few weeks to be sure any given drug is or is not useful.

Some articles document the existence of depressive and bipolar disorders manifesting somewhat atypically in relatively or completely nonverbal patients (Sovner 1986; Sovner and Hurley 1983). Such patients are appropriate candidates for treatment with standard antidepressants or lithium.

If one accepts that turbulent overactive assaultive behavior and episodically violent behavior toward others or self are usually not manifestations of psychosis in retarded patients or if it has been empirically determined that these are not neuroleptic-responsive behaviors, what then? Candidate drugs include lithium, buspirone, propranolol, nadolol, and carbamazepine. None of these have been the subject of placebo-controlled clinical trials in disturbed retarded patients, but all have been the subject of small open trials with reported sustained, often delayed, benefit in the patients described.

Lithium carbonate has the best credential as an antianger drug in a variety of psychiatric populations and should probably be tried first. If the patient has a seizure disorder, shifting to carbamazepine seems sensible. Nadolol is of theoretical interest because it is a beta-blocker that does not cross the blood-brain barrier, and it is hypothesized to decrease episodic violence by peripheral action on muscles. Propranolol requires more titrating (30–480 mg a day) to determine an effective dosage and can cause hypotension, bradycardia, and delirium. The desirable monitoring of vital signs before each dose above 120 mg a day may be impossible in some residential facilities.

Buspirone has been useful in doses of 15–60 mg a day, but onset of clinical action appears to be delayed. Local experts inform us that buspirone is less useful in the more violent retarded patient. Preliminary data suggest that fluoxetine may be effective in such patients. Further discussion of many of these drugs is found in Chapters 3–5.

In retarded or nonretarded patients with a seizure disorder, there is a worry that psychiatric drugs, including TCAs and neuroleptics, may lower the seizure threshold and increase the likelihood or rate of convulsions. There is no firm evidence that this, in fact, occurs. Maprotiline, imipramine, and amitriptyline have been more often connected with seizure occurrence in nonretarded depressed patients in our experience, but these were also the most commonly used tricyclics in the McLean Hospital system at the time seizures were seen. Trazodone is least likely to affect seizure threshold. Bupropion and clomipramine have also been associated with seizures. Among the neuroleptics there is a belief that haloperidol or molindone is least likely to affect seizure occurrence. In our experience, chlorpromazine and loxapine are occasionally associated with seizures. Seizures are more of a problem with clozapine (see Chapter 4).

In patients with a known seizure disorder that is adequately treated with anticonvulsants, it is relatively unlikely that any of the standard psychiatric drugs will make a clinically important difference in seizure frequency. In retarded patients on phenytoin, phenobarbital, or primidone for seizure control, there is a real possibility that the seizure medication may be causing cognitive dysfunction. It may be worth shifting the patient to carbamazepine to see if the patient may function better on that relatively different medication.

Stimulants may also be worth a trial in hyperactive retarded patients who are under close clinical observation. Stimulants have the advantage of causing clear clinical effects (improvement or worsening) within a few hours or days of reaching an adequate dose so that the trials of a stimulant may be completed in 1 or 2 weeks.

MEDICAL CONDITIONS

Some psychiatric syndromes are caused by or strongly associated with medical disorders. Others are commonly associated with medications used to treat medical or neurological conditions. On the other hand, some medical conditions and some drugs used to treat medical conditions complicate the use of standard psychoactive drugs to treat coexisting psychiatric disorders.

Psychiatric Disorders Resulting From Medical Illness

Psychiatric disorders, especially depression, can occur with and are presumably caused by thyroid or adrenal cortical dysfunction, uremia, cancer of the pancreas, and any metastatic carcinomatosis sufficiently often to make it worth ascertaining whether these conditions exist in depressed patients. Other more obvious conditions such as strokes, multiple sclerosis, lupus erythematosus, and Parkinson's disease are often associated with depression, as well as with organic brain dysfunction. Chronic pain syndromes including headache and low-back pain are so confounded with depressive syndromes that primary antidepressant therapy is often indicated and often effective. For some medical conditions such as hypothyroidism, treating the underlying condition is the first order of business. For others, the presence of an untreatable medical or neurological condition does not contraindicate, per se, standard antidepressant therapy.

Hyperthyroidism, caffeinism, hypoglycemia, temporal lobe epilepsy, paroxysmal tachycardias, and pheochromocytoma can all mimic panic disorder and should be ruled out. A medical reevaluation is indicated if standard drug therapies fail.

A recent review by Raj and Sheehan (1988) suggests some useful tips for making such key differential diagnoses. For example, attacks of paroxysmal atrial tachycardia generally begin and end more abruptly than do panic attacks and produce heart rates of 140–200 beats/minute. In contrast, heart rates in panic disorder rarely exceed 140 beats/minute. In pheochromocytoma, anxiety is only the fourth most common symptom, and many patients with this condition experience tachycardia and increased blood pressure without becoming unduly fearful. There is often an increased familial prevalence of neurofibromatosis and café au lait spots. Hyperthyroidism is associated with sleep disturbance, heat sensitivity, a more enduring tremor, etc. Finally, temporal lobe epilepsy may represent a more difficult diagnostic dilemma. In almost 25% of patients with this disorder, anxiety occurs during the aura. Such patients frequently, however, also complain of other symptoms—e.g., perceptual distortions and lapses of concentration. In assessing patients with possible panic disorder, a routine medical history and physical examination should be obtained. Laboratory tests should be ordered as needed to rule out specifically suspected conditions.

There is now a growing series of very positive case reports on the use of stimulants, mainly methylphenidate in doses of 10 mg once or twice a day, in patients with serious medical or surgical illnesses on medical services. These patients are noted on psychiatric consultation to be depressed, retarded, even almost mute, losing weight, not eating, unable to cooperate in treatment, withdrawn, and hopeless. Stimulants can produce relief in a day or two and can often be discontinued in 2–4 weeks, once the patient is generally improving. Of the 17 such case reports, none describe any serious side effects. By inference, elevated pulse or blood pressure is not a problem. Despite the appetite-reducing effect of stimulants in overweight subjects, these medically ill patients rapidly regain weight on methylphenidate. Sometimes stimulants are used because tricyclics are contraindicated, but the results are positive enough for stimulants to be considered first-choice drugs in these patients. Standard antidepressants rarely improve mood or functioning in a few days.

Depression following stroke has received some special study in recent years. It is clear that depression following cerebrovascular accidents occurs in about half the patients affected and can be relieved by antidepressants. There have been two controlled studies, one of nortriptyline and one of trazodone. Nortriptyline was generally effective, but 3 of the 17 patients studied developed delirium. Patients treated with medication longer and those with plasma levels over 100 ng/ml did better. Trazodone was less effective relative to placebo, but significant positive effects were found in dexamethasone nonsuppressors and patients with higher levels of depressive symptomatology. Slow cautious dosage increases are best with both drugs to avoid adverse effects. ECT has also been reported to be effective in poststroke depression. Most patients with cognitive impairment before ECT had improved cognitive functioning after ECT.

Psychiatric Disorders Associated With Medical Drugs

A variety of antihypertensive drugs (e.g., propranolol, reserpine, alpha-methyl-dopa) can sometimes precipitate depression. Shifting to a thiazide diuretic or a different, noncentrally acting beta-blocker (e.g., atenolol) can be helpful, or a TCA alone can sometimes adequately treat both the depression and the hypertension.

Diazepam has also occasionally been associated with increased depression. Both benzodiazepines and barbiturates can aggravate ADHD. Benzodiazepines may produce memory problems, particularly in—but not limited to—the elderly. Stimulants can aggravate schizophrenia or mania.

Steroids and L-dopa can mimic almost any known psychiatric syndrome including delirium, paranoid psychosis, mania, depression, and anxiety.

The whole range of drugs used in Parkinson's disease can cause hallucinosis and confusion. Sometimes anticholinergic drugs used in gastrointestinal disorders can also cause anticholinergic confusion and delirium, as can digitalis-like drugs and cimetidine-like agents.

It is impossible to list or predict all the drugs or drug combinations that at some dose in some patient can elicit or aggravate symptoms of psychiatric disorder. In patients receiving several drugs for medical conditions who present with depression, anxiety, or psychosis coming on after the drugs were begun, a careful reevaluation of the patient's pharmacotherapies is necessary. Stopping the less obviously crucial medications and shifting to less centrally active alternative drugs, where some medication is necessary, are reasonable steps.

Psychiatric Disorders Complicated by Medical Disorders

Many medical disorders could have reasonably predictable effects on the pharmacokinetics of standard psychiatric drugs, but the transition from theoretical data to practical application is often not exact. In the case of kidney failure and lithium therapy, the facts are clear. If renal clearance is decreased, lithium excretion will be decreased in a reasonably proportionate manner. In patients with substantially elevated serum creatinine and blood urea nitrogen who are not in acute renal failure, very small doses of lithium (e.g., 150 mg a day) can be cautiously begun and titrated in the same way as in a healthy patient, but more cautiously and with smaller increments. Here lithium citrate given in milliliter doses could give extra flexibility. We have heard of patients on renal dialysis who were stabilized on lithium by having a single 300-mg dose given after each episode of dialysis. This dose maintained an adequate blood level until the next dialysis removed the lithium ions.

With liver damage, the effects are more complicated. Most drugs are partially destroyed in the liver after absorption from the small intestine (the first-pass effect). When liver tissue is damaged, many drugs will get into the general circulation at much higher levels. Usually glucuronidation as a method of drug deactivation is well preserved, whereas demethylation and other metabolic processes are more readily impaired. This is why drugs like diazepam, which need to be demethylated, cause much higher blood levels per unit dose in cirrhosis, whereas drugs like lorazepam, which are only glucuronidated, are handled normally. Unfortunately, it is not always clear to even a skilled clinical pharmacologist exactly what the effect of chronic liver disease on the clinical actions of any particular drug will be. It is likely that standard tricyclics such as amitriptyline and imipramine will be less readily converted to their desmethyl metabolites, nortriptyline or desipramine, in patients with partial liver failure. The consequences of this shift—perhaps more sedation, confusion, or anticholinergic side effects—are less clear. The obvious lesson is to proceed very cautiously, to use blood level determinations, if available, and to assume that liver damage will markedly increase a drug's half-life, making gradual accumulation of higher and higher blood levels quite possible over a couple of weeks at a constant daily dose. Lowered blood protein levels, common in liver disease, may also increase free-drug levels, unbound to protein, making a drug more potent at lower total blood levels measured in the conventional manner.

An "overactive" liver can also pose problems. Some known drugs, including barbiturates, phenytoin, carbamazepine, and cigarette smoking, will induce hepatic enzymes and will increase the rate at which some psychiatric drugs are destroyed, making higher dosages necessary to achieve clinical results (see Chapters 3, 5, and 9). It is also worth noting that even drug-free patients can show large degrees of biological variability in their natural rates of drug metabolism. As an example, Glassman et al. (1977; in Chapter 3) found imipramine levels to vary from 40 to 1,040 ng/ml in depressed patients receiving 2.5 mg/kg of imipramine. Again, the lesson is that patients on other drugs for medical reasons may well have altered response, based either on increased or decreased hepatic metabolism of the psychiatric drug that has just been added (not to mention pharmacologic interactions such as additive sedation or additive postural hypotension). In the likely absence of clear knowledge as to the interactions in a particular patient of, say, cimetidine, phenytoin, chlorthiazide, and isoniazid with imipramine, the clinician adding imipramine in a patient on all these other drugs must be prepared to proceed cautiously but to use high dosages of imipramine if neither side effects nor clinical response occurs, if blood levels are low, and if ECG changes are not seen.

In cardiac patients there has long been a fear that all TCAs are cardiotoxic and likely to cause disastrous arrhythmias. Although they produce mild tachycardia (increase of 10 beats/minute) in medically healthy depressed patients, their arrhythmogenic potential appears to occur primarily if the drugs are taken in overdose. The mechanism by which the tricyclics and maprotiline affect cardiac function is a quinidine-like slowing of cardiac conduction. Tricyclics have, in fact, an ability to decrease cardiac irritability and suppress premature contractions. They are therefore *not* contraindicated in ordinary dosages in depressed patients with premature ventricular contractions and may well help both the cardiac irritability and the depression. The tricyclics should, however, be used with caution in patients with preexisting conduction defects, such as bundle-branch block. Patients with first-degree block have a 9% rate of 2:1 atrioventricular block development when on TCAs compared to a 0.7% rate in patients without first-degree block. Tricyclics should not be given to patients already on cardiac antiarrhythmic drugs, which act by slowing cardiac conduction, because additive effects on conduction could be harmful. Not all cardiologists are aware of the cardiac effects of tricyclics, and the psychiatrist who collaborates with cardiologists or primary-care physicians may need to do some educating of his or her consultants.

The other antidepressant with a possible effect on cardiac irritability is trazodone. It does not affect conduction but has occasionally, not regularly, been associated with an increase in premature ventricular contractions and should be avoided in patients with runs of PVCs or ventricular bigeminies. MAOIs, in therapeutic dosages, do not have obvious direct effects on cardiac conduction.

The serotonin reuptake blockers appear to produce a mild 3 beat/minute decrease in heart rate in medically healthy depressed patients. Although these agents have not yet been widely studied in post–myocardial infarction patients, their possible use in such patients is suggested by animal studies and by data available in cardiovascularly healthy depressive patients. In addition, these agents produce milder alterations in blood pressure than do other antidepressants.

The more significant effect of TCAs and MAOIs is postural hypotension, which can be aggravated (potentiated) in patients already on drugs such as propranolol, which are likely to cause hypotension as well. Although patients who have stable cardiac disease but are not in congestive failure probably tolerate antidepressants well, patients on multiple cardiac drugs are particularly prone to postural hypotension and other cardiac side effects. For seriously ill cardiac patients with severe depression, ECT may be the treatment of choice.

Bupropion has been assessed in depressed patients with moderate cardiac disease and seems to be better tolerated than the tricyclics, even nortriptyline. As indicated above, fluoxetine appears to have fewer negative effects on cardiac function and may also be better tolerated. Its potential for elevating tricyclic blood levels makes it worth warning the cardiologist to carefully monitor blood levels of cardiac drugs if fluoxetine is added to an already complex drug regimen in cardiac patients.

There is increasing evidence that depression in cardiac patients increases their mortality rate over time. The reasonable inference is that treating depression in cardiac patients, despite the problems noted above, is worthwhile. The clinician should, however, start with low drug dosages and proceed cautiously upward, monitoring blood levels and cardiac function carefully.

Another predictable interaction between psychiatric and general medical drugs is the additive effects of anticholinergic agents such as propantheline (Pro-Banthine), glycopyrrolate (Robinul), or preparations like Donnatal, which contain atropine and scopolamine as well as phenobarbital, or tincture of belladonna. It is possible that adding a potent anticholinergic, such as amitriptyline, to anticholinergic antispasmodics could result in urinary retention or paralytic ileus. Additive central anticholinergic effects could cause confusion or delirium. Here glycopyrrolate, which does not cross the blood-brain barrier, would be preferred to atropine if both an anticholinergic tricyclic and an anticholinergic antispasmodic were really needed at the same time.

Another serious, well-publicized interaction is the lethal potential of meperidine-MAOI combinations. However, many surgeons and internists still are unaware of this problem. In any patient on maintenance MAOI therapy being admitted to a hospital or an emergency room with pain or about to have major surgery, the psychiatrist should warn the treating doctor not to use meperidine. Morphine and codeine appear well tolerated, but the dosage should initially be low and increased only if no adverse effects occur. General anesthesia in patients on MAOIs can be used safely. If hypotension occurs during surgery, volume expanders are preferable to pressor drugs to avoid hypertensive crises.

Other additive or antagonistic interactions probably occur.

Some of the better-documented ones are discussed in earlier chapters focusing on specific drug classes.

It would be helpful if our current knowledge of drug actions could be put to precise clinical use in assessing the effects of adding a new psychiatric drug to a preexisting melange of medical and psychiatric drugs. Unfortunately, drugs do not work like sums in an algebraic equation. One would think, for example, that d-amphetamine, an indirect dopamine agonist, would have its action opposed by haloperidol, a reasonably pure dopamine blocking drug. In practice some patients will feel more lively and functional when d-amphetamine is added to haloperidol without becoming more psychotic. In practice, drugs usually act on several receptors and on both pre- and postsynaptic receptors of a single type, leading to potentially complex effects and interactions. The clinician is often faced with treating, say, schizophrenia, agoraphobia with panic, or depression in a patient with several medical problems that require concomitant drug therapies likely to influence the metabolism or absorption of a psychiatric drug or to have additive or antagonistic or, more likely, unknown effects in combination with the most appropriate psychiatric drug treatment. All drug therapy consists of a series of empirical clinical trials; medically ill patients simply present more complicated empirical trials. The psychiatrist can try to guess at the more probable ways in which the new drug will act or be affected by the patient's medical disease and ongoing drug therapies, but it is likely to be only guesswork. If there are semipredictable adverse interactions, one can try to either avoid them by choosing the psychiatric drug least likely to cause trouble or proceed cautiously with close monitoring of the patient for predictable and unpredictable side effects in collaboration with the physicians managing the patient's nonpsychiatric disorders. One worries that medically ill patients will be very fragile and easily become toxic on psychiatric drugs, but it is likely that this is not a general problem—some patients may develop problems, whereas others will tolerate psychiatric drugs unusually well. The reported use of huge haloperidol doses (e.g., 10 mg iv every hour for many hours) in medical or surgical intensive care units makes one wonder whether some seriously ill patients may not be exceedingly tolerant of some psychiatric drugs.

Bibliography

Ananth J: Side effects in the neonate from psychotropic agents excreted through breast feeding. Am J Psychiatry 135:801–805, 1978

Barkley R, Cunningham L: Do stimulant drugs improve academic performance of hyperkinetic children? a review of outcome studies. Clin Pediatr (Phila) 17:85–92, 1978

Bernstein JG: Drug interactions, in Massachusetts General Hospital Handbook of General Hospital Psychiatry, 3rd Edition. Chicago, IL, Mosby Yearbook (in press)

Breunning SE, Ferguson DG, Davidson NA, et al: Effects of thioridazine on the intellectual performance of mentally retarded drug responders and non-responders. Arch Gen Psychiatry 40:309–313, 1983

Briggs G, Bodendorfer T, Freeman R, et al: Drugs in Pregnancy and Lactation: A Reference Guide to Fetal and Neonatal Risk. Baltimore, MD, Williams & Wilkins, 1983

Campell M: Psychopharmacology in childhood psychosis. International Journal of Mental Health 4:238–254, 1975

Campbell M: Psychopharmacology, in Basic Handbook of Child Psychiatry. Edited by Noshpitz J, Harrison S. New York, Basic Books, 1979, pp 376–409

Campbell M: Drug treatment of infantile autism: the past decade, in Psychopharmacology: The Third Generation of Progress. Edited by Meltzer HY. New York, Raven, 1987, pp 1225–1232

Campbell M, Spencer E: Psychopharmacology in child and adolescent psychiatry: a review of past five years. J Am Acad Child Adolesc Psychiatry 27:269–279, 1988

Cohen B, Sommer B: Metabolism of thioridazine in the elderly . J Clin Psychopharmacol 8:336–339, 1988

Cohen DJ, Detlor J, Young JG, et al: Clonidine ameliorates Gilles de la Tourette's syndrome. Arch Gen Psychiatry 37:1350–1357, 1980

Cohen LS, Heller VL, Rosenbaum JF: Treatment guidelines for psychotropic drug use in pregnancy. Psychosomatics 30:25–33, 1989

Cole JO: Research issues, in Anxiety in the Elderly. Edited by Salzman C, Lebowitz BD. New York, Springer, 1990

Cole J, Hardy P, Marcel B, et al: Organic states, in Common Treatment Problems in Depression. Edited by Schatzberg A. Washington, DC, American Psychiatric Press, 1985, pp 79–100

Creasey W: Drug disposition in humans. New York, Oxford University Press, 1979

DeLong GR, Nieman GW: Lithium-induced behavior changes in children with symptoms suggesting manic-depressive illness. Psychopharmacol Bull 19:258–265, 1983

DiGiacomo J: The hypertensive or cardiac patient, in Common Treatment Problems in Depression. Edited by Schatzberg A. Washington, DC, American Psychiatric Press, 1985, pp 29–56

Eisendorfer C, Fann WE (eds): Psychopharmacology and Aging. New York, Plenum, 1973

Federoff JP, Robinson RG: Tricyclic antidepressants in the treatment of poststroke depression. J Clin Psychiatry 50 (suppl 7):18–23, 1989

Friedel R: Pharmacokinetics in the geropsychiatric patient, in Psychopharmacology: A Generation of Progress. Edited by Lipton M, DiMascio A, Killam K. New York, Raven, 1978, pp 1499–1506

Gastfriend DR, Biederman J, Jellinek MS: Desipramine in the treatment of adolescents with attention deficit disorders. Am J Psychiatry 141:906–908, 1984

Georgotas A, McCue R, Cooper T: A placebo-controlled comparison of nortriptyline and phenelzine in maintenance therapy of elderly depressed patients. Arch Gen Psychiatry 46:783–786, 1989

Gittelman-Klein R, Klein DF: Controlled imipramine treatment of school phobia. Arch Gen Psychiatry 25:204–207, 1971

Glassman A: The newer antidepressant drugs and their cardiovascular effects. Psychopharmacol Bull 20:272–277, 1984

Glassman A, Walsh B, Roose S, et al: Factors related to orthostatic hypotension associated with tricyclic antidepressants. J Clin Psychiatry 43:35–40, 1982

Gold M, Estroff T, Pottash A: Substance-induced organic mental disorders, in Psychiatry Update: American Psychiatric Association Annual Review, Vol 4. Edited by Hales RE, Frances AJ. Washington, DC, American Psychiatric Press, 1985, pp 227–240

Goldberg H, DiMascio A: Psychotropic drugs in pregnancy, in Psychopharmacology: A Generation of Progress. Edited by Lipton M, DiMascio A, Killam K. New York, Raven, 1978, pp 1047–1055

Greenblatt D, Shader R: Psychotropic drugs in the general hospital, in Manual of Psychiatric Therapeutics. Edited by Shader R. Boston, MA, Little, Brown, 1975, pp 1–26

Gualtieri CT, Barnhill J, McGimsey J, et al: Tardive dyskinesia and other movement disorders in children treated with psychotropic drugs. J Am Acad Child Psychiatry 19:491–510, 1980

Helms PM: Efficacy of antipsychotics in the treatment of the behavioral complications of dementia: a review of the literature. J Am Geriatr Soc 33:206–209, 1985

Huessey H, Ruoff P: Towards a rational drug usage in a state institution for retarded individuals. Psychiatr J Univ Ottawa 9:56–58, 1984

Leonard H, Swedo S, Rapoport J: Treatment of obsessive-compulsive disorder with clomipramine and desipramine in children and adolescents: a double-blind crossover comparison. Arch Gen Psychiatry 46:1088–1092, 1989

Lipsey J, Robinson R, Pearlsen J, et al: Nortriptyline treatment of post-stroke depression. Lancet 1:297–300, 1984

Mikkelsen E, Rapoport J: Enuresis: psychopathology, sleep stage and drug response. Urol Clin North Am 1:361–375, 1980

Morgan MH, Read AE: Antidepressants and liver disease. Gut 13:697–701, 1972

Paykel E, Fleminger R, Watson J: Psychiatric side effects of antihypertensive drugs. J Clin Psychopharmacol 2:14–33, 1982

Petti T, Law W: Imipramine treatment of depressed children: a double-blind pilot study. J Clin Psychopharmacol 2:107–110, 1982

Platt JE, Campbell M, Green WH, et al: Cognitive effects of lithium carbonate and haloperidol in treatment-resistant aggressive children. Arch Gen Psychiatry 41:657–662, 1984

Popper CW: Child and adolescent psychopharmacology, in Psychiatry. Edited by Michaels R, Cavenar JO, Brodie HK, et al. Philadelphia, PA, Lippincott, 1985, pp 1138–1159

Popper C, Famularo R: Child and adolescent psychopharmacology, in Developmental-Behavioral Pediatrics. Edited by Levine MD, Carey WB, Crocker AC, et al. Philadelphia, PA, WB Saunders, 1983

Prien RF: Chemotherapy in chronic organic brain syndrome: a review of the literature. Psychopharmacol Bull 9:5–20, 1973

Raj AB, Sheehan DV: Medical evaluation of the anxious patient. Psychiatric Annals 18:176–181, 1988

Raskin DE: Antipsychotic medications and the elderly. J Clin Psychiatry 46 (no 5, sec 2):36–40, 1985

Ratey JJ, Sovner R, Mikkelsen E, et al: Buspirone therapy for maladaptive behavior and anxiety in developmentally disabled persons. J Clin Psychiatry 50:382–384, 1989

Ray WA, Griffin MR, Schaffner W, et al: Psychotropic drug use and the risk of hip fracture. N Engl J Med 316:363–369, 1987

Ray WA, Griffin MR, Downey W: Benzodiazepines of long and short elimination half-life and the risk of hip fracture. JAMA 262:3303–3307, 1989

Reisberg B, Ferris SH, Gershon S: An overview of pharmacologic treatment of cognitive decline in the elderly. Am J Psychiatry 138:593–600, 1981

Salzman CA: A primer of geriatric psychopharmacology. Am J Psychiatry 139:67–74, 1982

Salzman CA: Practical considerations in the pharmacologic treatment of depression and anxiety in the elderly. J Clin Psychiatry 51 (suppl 1):21–26, 1990

Schaerf FW, Miller RR, Lipsey JR, et al: ECT for major depression in four patients infected with human immunodeficiency virus. Am J Psychiatry 146:782–784, 1989

Schiffer RB, Herndon RM, Rudick RA: Treatment of pathologic laughing and weeping with amitriptyline. N Engl J Med 312:1480–1482, 1985

Shader RI (ed): Psychiatric Complications of Medical Drugs. New York, Raven, 1972

Shapiro AK, Shapiro E, Wayne H: Treatment of Tourette's syndrome. Arch Gen Psychiatry 28:92–97, 1973

Shepard TH: The Catalogue of Teratogenic Agents, 4th Edition. Baltimore, MD, Johns Hopkins University Press, 1983

Silver J, Hales R, Yudofsky S: Psychopharmacology of depression in neurologic disorders. J Clin Psychiatry 51 (suppl 1):33–39, 1990

Sovner R: Limiting factors in the use of DSM-III criteria with mentally ill/mentally retarded patients. Psychopharmacol Bull 22:1055–1059, 1986

Sovner R: The use of valproate in the treatment of mentally retarded persons with typical and atypical bipolar disorders. J Clin Psychiatry 50:40(S)–43(S), 1989

Sovner R, Hurley A: Do the mentally retarded suffer from affective illness? Arch Gen Psychiatry 40:61–67, 1983

Summers W, Majovski L, Marsh G, et al: Oral tetrahydroaminoacridine in long term treatment of senile dementia. N Engl J Med 315:1241–1245, 1986

Thompson TL, Moran MG, Nies AS: Psychotropic drug use in the elderly (Part 2). N Engl J Med 308:194–199, 1985

Tinetti ME, Speechley M: Prevention of falls among the elderly. N Engl J Med 320:1055–1059, 1989

Tsuang MM, Lu L, Stotsky BA, et al: Haloperidol vs thioridazine for hospitalized psychogeriatric patients: double-blind study. J Am Geriatr Soc 19:593–600, 1971

Werry JS (ed): Pediatric Psychopharmacology. New York, Brunner/Mazel, 1978

Wragg RE, Jeste DV: Neuroleptics and alternative treatments: management of behavioral symptoms and psychosis in Alzheimer's disease and related conditions. Psychiatr Clin North Am 11:195–213, 1988

Wragg R, Jeste D: Overview of depression and psychosis in Alzheimer's disease. Am J Psychiatry 146:577–587, 1989

Yudofsky SC, Silver JM, Schneider SE: The use of beta blockers in the treatment of aggression. Psychiatry Letters 6:15–23, 1988

Appendix

Strengths and costs per 100 pills of antidepressant drugs

Drug	Strength (mg)	Cost per 100 pills*
amitriptyline	25	$ 4
desipramine	25	21
doxepin	25	11
imipramine	25	4
nortriptyline	25	42
protriptyline	10	50
trimipramine	25	24
amoxapine	25	40
maprotiline	25	27
bupropion	100	48
clomipramine	50	85
fluoxetine	20	132
isocarboxazid	10	36
phenelzine	15	20
tranylcypromine	10	25
trazodone	50	18
acetophenazine	20	32
chlorpromazine	100	5
chlorprothixene	100	58
fluphenazine	2.5	50
haloperidol	2	20
loxapine	10	55
mesoridazine	50	43
molindone	10	36
perphenazine	8	50
pimozide	2	45
thioridazine	100	18
thiothixene	5	21
trifluoperazine	5	10
clozapine	50	172/wk

* Cost is reported as the average wholesale price (AWP) based on the 1989 Redbook.

Suggested Reading List

For Clinicians

American Psychiatric Association: Benzodiazepine Dependence, Toxicity, and Abuse: A Task Force Report of the American Psychiatric Association. Washington, DC, American Psychiatric Association, 1990

Baldessarini RJ: Biomedical Aspects of Depression and Its Treatment. Washington, DC, American Psychiatric Press, 1983

Baldessarini RJ: Chemotherapy in Psychiatry: Principles and Practice. Cambridge, MA, Harvard University Press, 1985

Cole JO (ed): Psychopharmacology Update. Lexington, MA, Collamore Press, 1980

Gilman AG, Goodman LS, Gilman A (eds): Goodman and Gilman's The Pharmacological Basis of Therapeutics, 8th Edition. New York, Pergamon, 1990

Hyman SE (ed): Manual of Psychiatric Emergencies. Boston, MA, Little, Brown, 1984

Jefferson JW, Greist JH, Ackerman DL, et al: Lithium Encyclopedia for Clinical Practice, 2nd Edition. Washington, DC, American Psychiatric Press, 1986

Klein DF, Davis JM: Diagnosis and Drug Treatment of Psychiatric Disorders. Baltimore, MD, Williams & Wilkins, 1969

Klein DF, Gittelman-Klein R, Quitkin F, et al: Diagnosis and Drug Treatment of Psychiatric Disorders: Adults and Children. Baltimore, MD, Williams & Wilkins, 1980

Mason AS, Granacher RPL: Clinical Handbook of Antipsychotic Drug Therapy. New York, Brunnel/Mazel, 1980

McElroy SL, Pope HG Jr: Use of Anticonvulsants in Psychiatry: Recent Advances. Clifton, NJ, Oxford Health Care, 1988

Meltzer HY (ed): Psychopharmacology: The Third Generation of Progress. New York, Raven, 1987

Tupin JP, Shader RI, Harnett DS (eds): Handbook of Clinical Psychopharmacology, 2nd Edition. Northvale, NJ, Jason Aronson, 1988

For Patients and Families

Andreasen NC: The Broken Brain: The Biological Revolution in Psychiatry. New York, Harper & Row, 1984

Burns D: The Feeling Good Handbook. New York, William Morrow, 1989

Fieve RR: Moodswing: The Third Revolution in Psychiatry. New York, Bantam, 1976

Gold MS: The Good News About Panic, Anxiety, and Phobias. New York, Villard, 1989

Klein DF, Wender PH: Do You Have a Depressive Illness? How to Tell, What to Do. New York, New American Library, 1988

Kline NS: From Sad to Glad. New York, Ballantine, 1981

Korpell HS: How You Can Help: A Guide for Families of Psychiatric Hospital Patients. Washington, DC, American Psychiatric Press, 1984

Mendelson JH, Mello NK: Alcohol Use and Abuse in America. Boston, MA, Little, Brown, 1985

Pope HG, Hudson JI: New Hope for Binge Eaters. New York, Harper & Row, 1984

Schou M: Lithium Treatment of Manic-Depressive Illness, 2nd Edition. Basel, Karger, 1983

Sheehan DV: The Anxiety Disease and How to Overcome It. New York, Scribner, 1984

Stone EM (ed): American Psychiatric Glossary, 6th Edition. Washington, DC, American Psychiatric Press, 1988

Styron W: Darkness Visible: A Memoir of Madness. New York, Random House, 1990

Tsuang MT: Schizophrenia: The Facts. New York, Oxford University Press, 1982

Winokur G: Depression: The Facts. New York, Oxford University Press, 1981

Index

All page numbers in bold italic type refer to tables or figures in the text.

I